MOLD ILLNESS:

SURVIVING AND THRIVING

A RECOVERY MANUAL FOR PATIENTS & FAMILIES IMPACTED BY CIRS

PAULA VETTER, RN, MSN, FNP-C

LAURIE ROSSI, RN

CINDY EDWARDS, CBA

DEDICATION

This manual is dedicated to Dr. Ritchie Shoemaker, the visionary pioneer who identified and tirelessly unraveled the mysteries of the previously elusive syndrome, now known as CIRS.

Dr. Shoemaker's relentless dedication to rigorous scientific investigation and documentation produced a protocol that has empowered thousands of patients to reclaim their lives.

The Surviving and Thriving Recovery Manual is a tribute to the living legacy of Dr. Shoemaker.

This manual is also dedicated to the struggles of countless thousands of CIRS patients, many still undiagnosed. Here you will find a voice, a beacon of hope, and a roadmap to recovery. You are not alone.

TESTIMONIALS FROM CIRS PATIENTS

In working with Paula and Laurie, I was taught about the physiology of CIRS…..what was happening to my body and how we were going to reverse these devastating effects. I had never had medical treatment like this before. Someone actually cared enough about me to teach me to be my own advocate going forward. I now had the tools to manage CIRS.

When I got the results of my home and work mold tests, Laurie and Paula put me in touch with Cindy Edwards, an amazing CIRS literate environmental professional and certified building analyst. Cindy was able to walk me through the details of what I needed to do to make my environments safe for me. All of this was a tremendous amount of work but my "team" was there for me every step of the way. They gave me encouragement and even tough love when I needed it. They even helped to educate my local primary care doctor so that she could provide the appropriate follow-up care for me and for others with CIRS.

*It has been a little over four years since I first became sick. I am finishing up my VIP and feeling better than I have in longer than I can remember. All of my blood work is slowly improving and I am finally feeling hopeful about my future again thanks to my partnership with this team of professionals. **K B***

Paula and Laurie provided me with comprehensive information and references to educate me about CIRS, its causes, and its multiple complex effects. Laurie taught a very thorough class to reinforce this learning and to teach us about how to get better through symptom tracking, the Shoemaker Protocol, and appropriate mold remediation in our homes and workplaces. Paula and Laurie scheduled periodic appointments with me to keep track of biomarkers and help me with each step of the protocol. Cindy Edwards, my home performance and biotoxin specialist, consulted with me on a regular basis about how to make sure that my home was safe for me and my family.

I am now a good way through the protocol. I am grateful to them for their knowledge, professionalism, accessibility, and conscientiousness. This is such a difficult and complicated disease that I could never have navigated treatment on my own with my primary care physician.

Most of all, I am grateful to Paula, Laurie, and Cindy for their kindness, empathy, and integrity. They care deeply about their patients and want them to get better. They invited questions and answered all I had with plentiful information and references to resources, and treated me with respect. This team has helped me get better so that I will be able to live a full life, and I will never forget that. **PD**

TABLE OF CONTENTS

APPENDIX

INTRODUCTION

It is with great pleasure that I write to introduce the world to the dedication of Paula Vetter, FNP-C, Laurie Rossi, RN, and Cindy Edwards, C.B.A. They have been working as a team for several years to distill thousands of pages of academic material on all aspects of diagnosis and treatment of chronic inflammatory response syndrome (CIRS) into a short, concise, reader-accessible manual. This publication belongs on the desk of every physician who sees patients with CIRS, every patient who has concerns about a multi-system, multi-symptom illness, and anyone who lives, works or goes to school in the interior environment of a water-damaged building (WDB).

The blunt facts are that CIRS is incredibly common in today's American society. Back in 2011, the National Institute for Occupational Safety and Health published their opinions that suggested that as many as 50% of US buildings were water-damaged. 50% seems low based on surveys taken by thousands of patients.

Well, so what? Who needs a manual about treatment? WDB never hurt a flea, much less a person, right? Nope. CIRS is one of the most compelling reasons for the explosion of CFS, fibromyalgia and "depression" seen in the US.

So many people ill from WDB? How can that be? The answer is simple: It is all based on inflammation that is rooted in innate immune responses to "foreign invaders," called antigens. The inside of a WDB is always a soup of antigens, with sources coming from microbes like fungi, actinomycetes and bacteria. Mycotoxins make up about 1% of the risk (not a typo. Mycotoxins are trivial in importance compared to actinomycetes and bacteria). Antigen detection leads to inflammation, with harmful gene activation just a moment away from innate immune inflammation.

If we assume that only half of the people in the US might have exposure to WDB that means that maybe 160 million people are at risk for development of CIRS. Since we know that only 25% of all patients have the genetic makeup (HLA haplotype) that can create increased relative risk (susceptibility) to the innate immune illness that is CIRS that means that 40 million people in the US could possibly have problems related to untreated innate immune inflammation.

What that number means is that we add up the number of patients with symptoms-only diagnoses like fibromyalgia, Chronic Fatigue Syndrome, Post Lyme syndrome, reflex sympathetic dystrophy, even depression, as well as Post Traumatic Stress Disorder, and many others we get about 40 million. There are real possibilities that the 40 million number of patients with untreated chronic inflammatory illness is right on the button.

If WDB adds to the problems of those with Post-Lyme, and that occurrence surely is true, the good news is that we have peer-reviewed published documentation of efficiency of a treatment protocol, which step by step will arbitrarily take about one month (each) to correct one abnormality followed by another of innate immune inflammation. Following this protocol gives physicians the ability to measure objective parameters each step along the way, verifying the time for the next step has arrived. We also have the capability to correct differential genomic activation (transcriptomics). Finally, we can show that use of this sequential protocol corrects multinuclear atrophy of grey matter structures in the brain.

These are stunning results.

A barrier to understanding CIRS and its application to treatment of complex illnesses requires learning a new jargon; requires learning a new language; and demands rigorous approaches to science where assumptions are not tolerated and only one step at a time is undertaken with monitoring of each step along the way. We don't permit guesses; we don't permit assumptions, we don't permit speculation. Follow the data!

How is a person supposed to understand this jargon, this new language? The answer is right in front of you. Paula Vetter working together with her colleagues, Laurie Rossi and Cindy Edwards, makes the complexity of language and the complexity of science come alive. Imagine making transcriptomics and antigen presentation easy to read!

I recommend anyone with an interest in never-ending, multi-symptom, multisystem illnesses, especially those acquired following exposure to the interior environment of WDB, to read and learn what these three authors have given to us.

This manual is a prize. This manual is indeed the living legacy of Paula, Laurie and Cindy.

Ritchie C. Shoemaker, MD
Pocomoke, Md

FOREWORD

Got Mold?

Tired? Get headaches? Muscle aches? Stomach issues? Lousy sleep? Urinate all the time? Is your brain a little foggy?

Doctors can't tell you what's wrong with you? Do all their treatments fail?

Then this book is for you!

40 million Americans suffer from CIRS (chronic inflammatory response syndrome). Repeated exposure to moldy buildings and other environmental exposures create seemingly unrelated symptoms all over the body. CIRS is a genetic illness causing chronic inflammation leading to decreased blood flow, leaky junctions, brain and gut inflammation and improper regulation of any system in the body. Most sufferers aren't even aware that there is a single illness that explains all of their symptoms. Many of their doctors aren't either!

Surviving and Thriving is the most concise yet comprehensive primer I have ever read on how to diagnose, how to treat, and most importantly, how to live with CIRS. The authors, Paula Vetter, Laurie Rossi, and Cindy Edwards, rely on their professional expertise, personal stories and private experience to convey a wealth of CIRS knowledge. No other tome explains the CIRS life in such a straightforward manner. This manual is a gem and should be read by every CIRS sufferer and their family members.

My own CIRS saga began in 2009. I was asked to draw blood tests on some sick children at a local high school. I evaluated and examined 14 children and a teacher who had spent significant time at that institution. Their stories were amazing and so very similar. They averaged 21 symptoms! Many of these children were 14 and 15 years old! Subsequent lab work demonstrated a flurry of abnormal blood tests relating to their innate immune systems and the regulation of critical body systems. They clearly had the same illness, but I didn't know what it was. Further investigation led me to Dr. Ritchie Shoemaker who had already studied CIRS, treated patients, and written about this illness for 12 years. Now, I have evaluated over 1200 patients, co-authored 9 peer reviewed publications and consensus statements, spoken at numerous national and international conferences and testified a number of times as an expert witness about CIRS. When a certification for CIRS became available, I was the first to certify. I am honored to have been asked to write the foreword for this amazing work.

In October of 2013, Laurie organized and hosted a CIRS conference in San Luis Obispo, CA (or SLO, as the natives call it). Dr. Shoemaker, myself, and 3 other speakers presented "Biotoxin Illness- The science behind accurate diagnosis and effective treatment." I met Laurie, Paula, and Cindy for the first time at this conference. I consider each of these three women to be extraordinary. Laurie is an R.N. and a recovering CIRS sufferer. She was so knowledgeable and so sincere. She poured her heart into that very successful meeting as she does with everything she touches. This book is no different. Everything she writes about, she has lived.

Cindy also attended the SLO conference. She provided my first in depth exposure to building performance. Her knowledge not only blew my mind, but took me much deeper into the understanding of the building envelope and just how many variables can create a water intrusion inside your home, your office building or your school.

Paula was in the SLO audience in October of 2013. She is a holistic nurse practitioner, with more than 30 years of experience in both traditional and holistic medicine. She was studying Dr. Shoemaker's protocol and in the process of certifying. After completing her certification with Dr. Shoemaker, she teamed up with Laurie and Cindy. Their unique multi-disciplinary clinical practice successfully treated and educated patients, prior to Paula's recent retirement.

Our paths have crossed several more times discussing patients, advances in CIRS, presenting at the first and second State of the Art CIRS conferences and another SLO meeting populated by local CIRS aficionados and some world class barbecued chicken pizza (mangia!)

Paula, Laurie, and Cindy have poured their varied experiences into this comprehensive manual. Each has personal and practical knowledge as a patient, as a practitioner, as a nurse, as healers, as mothers, as an indoor environmental expert, as wives and as compassionate people intensely aware of a terrible illness.

CIRS can be daunting to patients because the primary treatment is to avoid toxic environments. Perhaps 50% of buildings are considered water-damaged and can be toxic to a CIRS patient. How does one determine if their home is safe, find a new apartment or buy a house? How does one choose a school for their children with CIRS. How does one find a CIRS-knowledgeable doctor or explain the illness to family? What caveats are present with the medication protocol? How does one detect if a new building is water-damaged? All these and many more questions are answered in the following pages.

These three experts, in their own areas, take the CIRS newbie through every conceivable scenario and give outstanding advice. No more need for trial and very costly error. Their compilation of guidance will be useful for even seasoned CIRS subjects. All three women have been there and done that! They share their extraordinary comprehension of the life CIRS patients suffer. They can do so because they have walked the walk!

Every patient with CIRS, every family member of a CIRS sufferer, every landlord, every boss and every doctor should read this book. If you know someone who has many symptoms but no real answers or who has been told they have an illness for which we doctors have little information and ineffective treatments, you should read this book. If you are feeling more and more tired, achy, sleeping poorly, having headaches, urinating all the time and not thinking as clearly as you used to, you should read this book. CIRS is no joke, but all the information you need to not just survive, but to thrive, is in *Surviving and Thriving*!

Scott W. McMahon, MD
Founder, Whole World Health Care and The Joseph Foundation, LLC
CIRS expert, speaker and published researcher
Roswell, New Mexico

WHAT IS CHRONIC INFLAMMATORY RESPONSE SYNDROME?

"Mold Illness", medically known as Chronic Inflammatory Response Syndrome (CIRS), is a topic of great interest. There is an abundance of information on this subject, and MUCH of it is incorrect!

In many cases, misleading statements are made by well meaning individuals who simply do not understand the complexity of the disease. Occasionally, unscrupulous and ill-informed entrepreneurs are just eager to sell their wares to ill people who are desperate to get well.

Too many people with CIRS have wasted thousands of dollars, and precious time, on treatments based on speculation rather than science. This manual, based on the most current science, provides a detailed and validated roadmap to recovery. This collection of practical information and survival tools will help you make good decisions about your health and recovery on a daily basis.

Science is not static; it evolves with new knowledge and understanding. That knowledge needs to be constantly validated with meticulous care.

This manual was written with a single purpose: to educate and empower individuals and families affected by CIRS to take charge of their health and transform their lives.

The journey to recovery is not easy, but it is possible. The tools provided here make navigating the journey much clearer and simpler than ever before. It is important for you to know that **you are not alone**. There are scientifically PROVEN solutions that WORK! The missing piece of the puzzle, up until now, has been a simplified roadmap to recovery, a practical guide that focuses on the daily challenges faced by millions with "mold illness." This manual fills that gap.

NOTE: This manual does NOT replace the personalized guidance of a Certified CIRS Practitioner and a CIRS Literate Indoor Environmental Professional.

It is beyond the scope of this "Survival Manual" to provide detailed information about the complex physiology involved in CIRS. The **Resources & References** sections will direct you to a number of scientifically accurate and detailed explanations of this complex illness.

Definition of CIRS?
("Mold Illness" or "Biotoxin Illness")

The term "mold illness" is actually a biotoxin illness called **Chronic Inflammatory Response Syndrome** (**CIRS**). The official medical definition of CIRS is:

"An acute and chronic, systemic inflammatory response syndrome acquired following exposure to the interior environment of a water-damaged building with resident toxigenic organisms, including, but not limited to fungi, bacteria, actinomycetes and mycobacteria as well as inflammagens such as endotoxins, beta glucans, hemolysins, proteinases, mannans and possibly spirocyclic drimanes, as well as volatile organic compounds (VOC's)."

What does that mean in plain English?

The air in a water-damaged building (WDB) is contaminated by a "chemical soup" of molds, bacteria and associated chemicals. When a susceptible individual inhales this contaminated air, the innate immune system will be activated, causing severe inflammation throughout the body. (We will discuss a little later who those "susceptible individuals" are.)

NOTE: You can also develop CIRS from the toxins in a brown recluse spider bite, from tropical fish that have been contaminated with ciguatera toxin, from Pfiesteria and cyanobacteria, and from Borrelia burgdorferi, the organism responsible for Lyme disease. **Water-damaged buildings, however, are the cause for 80% of CIRS.**

Chronic Inflammatory Response Syndrome (CIRS) is a multi-system and multi-symptom disease. It is caused by generalized inflammation, triggered by an immune system "out of control." It is a legitimate medical diagnosis with specific lab tests and physical findings that verify the diagnosis. **25% of the population has the specific genetic makeup that makes them vulnerable to CIRS.**

Exposure to mold (dead or alive), mold fragments, mold by-products, and other inflammatory chemicals found in water-damaged buildings (WDB), will cause the immune system of a susceptible individual to release inflammatory chemical into the circulation. Inhaling microscopic mold fragments, and the associated toxins, triggers massive inflammation in the body (including the brain) of someone with CIRS.

Mold does not need to be visible to cause harm to the individual with CIRS. Microscopic particles of mold toxins, and associated inflammatory molecules can be inhaled from heating or air conditioning ducts, carpets, upholstered furniture, other contaminated home contents, and air drawn from wall spaces in tightly sealed buildings. (More about this in the environmental section.)

A mere 48 hours of dampness from a minor leak or water intrusion is enough to make carpet, drywall, furniture and other porous surfaces a dangerous reservoir of mold, mold fragments, bacteria and toxic mold by-products. It is estimated that 50% of buildings in the US have water damage.

NOTE: MUCH more information on the environmental aspects of CIRS to follow!

What CIRS is NOT:

CIRS is NOT an allergy to mold. It is NOT mold growing in your body.

CIRS is NOT "all in your head." Most importantly, **CIRS IS NOT BEYOND YOUR CONTROL**. It can be reliably diagnosed and effectively treated with the Shoemaker Protocol, already validated in more than 10,000 patients.

Certain molds are highly toxic, and may cause health issues for anyone, but CIRS is discriminating. This chronic inflammatory condition is confined, almost exclusively, to those with specific genetic profiles. (We will discuss how to determine if you have the genetic profile that makes you susceptible to CIRS a little later.)

HOW DO I KNOW IF I HAVE CIRS?

The diagnosis of CIRS relies on specific criteria:

1. History of exposure to WDB
2. A collection of specific symptoms (multi-system)
3. Specific lab test abnormalities (including genetic testing)
4. Specific physical exam findings
5. Improvement in symptoms and labs with specific treatment

Accurate diagnosis of CIRS is essential. The problem is that the specific tests that identify CIRS are not part of any "routine" screening. If CIRS is not on your practitioner's "radar", it will not be detected. Patients with CIRS are often misdiagnosed with fibromyalgia, chronic fatigue, depression, Stress, Allergy, MS, PTSD, IBS, ADD, dementia, and more!

Symptoms of Mold Exposure:

There are many, seemingly unrelated, symptoms, because CIRS causes widespread inflammation of multiple body systems, including the brain. Following are common symptoms seen in those with CIRS:

Fatigue, Weakness, Aches, Muscle Cramps, Unusual Pains, Ice Pick Pains, Headache, Light Sensitivity, Red Eyes, Blurred Vision, Tearing, Sinus Problems, Cough, Shortness of Breath, Abdominal Pain, Diarrhea, Joint Pain, Morning Stiffness, Difficulty Learning New Information, Confusion, Memory Problems, Poor Focus & Concentration, Skin Sensitivity, Mood Swings, Appetite Swings, Sweats (especially at night), Poor Temperature

Regulation, Excessive Thirst, Increased Urination, Static Shocks, Numbness, Tingling, Vertigo, Metallic Taste, Tremor

Your practitioner will take a detailed inventory of your symptoms as part of your evaluation. The 37 common symptoms have been grouped into a system of 13 Clusters, further improving the accuracy of the diagnosis. You will find the **Symptom/Cluster Analysis** in the Appendix.

NOTE: The Symptom/Cluster Analysis should be administered by a Certified CIRS Practitioner. Many of the symptoms are subtle. Crucial diagnostic information may be missed without with specific and detailed targeted questions, tailored to the individual patient.

Specific Testing for CIRS:

Individuals who experience a significant number of the multi-system symptoms above, should have initial objective testing to establish the diagnosis of CIRS. The Vision (VCS) tests and HLA-DR can be done prior to making an appointment with a Certified CIRS Specialist.

VISUAL CONTRAST SENSITIVITY (VCS) TEST

The VCS test is a measure of one of the neurologic functions of vision known as "contrast". Biotoxins impair the ability to detect subtle contrast within 24 - 36 hours after exposure. This test is an extremely valuable, yet under-utilized, tool to detect and monitor exposure to toxic environments for individuals with CIRS.

The online VCS screening test is convenient and affordable, and can be done anytime you question a potential exposure. The instructions must be followed carefully to provide valid results. The online test should be periodically confirmed with an in-office hand-held testing device, conducted by a certified CIRS Practitioner.

For either the online or in-office test, your corrected visual acuity must be better than 20/50. If you normally wear glasses, wear them for the screening test. Be consistent with this. There must be adequate illumination. We use a light meter to confirm 70 foot-lamberts or more. Light from both the illuminated computer screen and an overhead light is usually adequate.

The test is taken with one eye covered and one open at a distance of 18" from the computer screen. You will do the test first with the left eye and then with the right eye. You need to make sure the distance from the screen stays constant at 18". Cutting a string to a length of 18 inches helps to keep the distance correct.

Your score is recorded according to published criteria for VCS testing. It is a "Pass/Fail," though specific deficits can be used to track your improvement over time or worsening with re-exposure. When you take the VCS Test online, you will receive immediate results to share with your practitioner.

Remember that this under-utilized tool can be done inexpensively, online, ANYTIME you want to confirm or rule out biotoxin exposure. Used along with symptom and activity tracking, it will provide extremely valuable information to guide your journey to recovery.

LAB TESTING for CIRS:

The first lab test required is the **HLA-DR**. This test identifies the genetic susceptibility to CIRS. It is extremely rare to have CIRS-WDB if you do NOT have a susceptible gene. (Read more about HLA-DR under "Why Did I Get Sick.")

If the VCS test is failed, then an HLA-DR blood test should be performed to verify genetic susceptibility. This can be ordered by your Primary Care Practitioner (PCP), or in consultation with a Certified CIRS Practitioner. Additional lab tests for specific biomarkers, as well as appropriate tests for differential diagnosis, should be scheduled.

The specific labs used to diagnose and monitor the clinical progress in CIRS are listed below. It is important to know that these are NOT part of routine labs screening profiles. Unless your practitioner is specifically LOOKING for CIRS, these labs will not likely be ordered.

These biomarkers will help to confirm the diagnosis and also help in monitoring your progress with the treatment protocol.

Lab Tests (Biomarkers) for CIRS:
MSH - Melanocyte Stimulating Hormone Normal Range: 35-81 pg/mL

MSH has multiple anti-inflammatory and hormone regulating functions. MSH regulates the pituitary, often referred to as the "master gland."

More than 95% of patients with CIRS will have a low MSH. Without adequate MSH, there is increased susceptibility to mold toxins, ongoing fatigue, pain, hormone abnormalities, sleep disturbance, mood swings, brain fog and more. MSH controls many other hormones, inflammation pathways, and basic defenses against invading microbes. Low MSH leaves the gut and respiratory systems vulnerable to multiply antibiotic resistant coagulase negative staphylococcus (MARCoNS) and other microbial disruption.

TGF Beta-1 - Transforming Growth Factor Beta-1
Normal Range: <2380 pg/ml

TGF Beta-1 is a critical lab marker that has important regulatory effects throughout the innate immune system. This protein helps control the growth, division, differentiation and motility of cells. It also regulates the process of apoptosis, the normal process of orchestrated "cell death" that eliminates old or diseased cells in the body.

Elevated TGF Beta-1 causes fibrosis and "remodeling" in tissues. It is often responsible for nasal and vocal cord polyps, as well as fibrosis and thickening in the lungs. Neurologic, autoimmune and many other systemic problems also are found with high TGF Beta-1.

TGFB-1, when monitored carefully along with C4a, can be a reliable indicator of biotoxin burden. They will both increase with re-exposure to WDB and decrease with removal from exposure.

C4a Normal Range: 0-2830 ng/ml

C4a is an inflammatory marker of great significance. C4a reflects the innate immune responses in those with exposure to Water Damaged Buildings (WDB). It will be elevated within 12 hours of acute exposure. (In some patients, C4a will be suppressed by the presence of MARCoNS.)

The complement system is a group of proteins that move freely through your bloodstream. The proteins work with your immune system and play a role in the development of inflammation.

Each complement protein regulates inflammatory responses. These short-lived proteins are re-manufactured rapidly and a rise of plasma levels is seen within 4-12 hours of exposure to biotoxins. The elevation will persist until definitive therapy is initiated.

MMP-9 Normal Range: 85-332 ng/mL

Matrix metallopeptidase 9 (MMP-9) is an enzyme that is involved in the orderly breakdown of certain tissues in normal physiology, as well as in disease. Excess MMP-9 disrupts tissue within blood vessel walls and causes inflammation of the brain, lungs, muscles, peripheral nerves and joints.

It has the ability to wreak havoc in COPD, rheumatoid arthritis, atherosclerosis, cardiomyopathy, and abdominal aortic aneurysm by attacking cells indiscriminately.

VEGF Normal Range: 31-86 pg/mL

Vascular endothelial growth factor (VEGF) is a substance made by cells that stimulates the growth of new blood vessels and increases blood flow in the capillaries. This improves circulation, along with improved delivery of oxygen and nutrients to the body. Deficiency of VEGF is a common and quite serious problem in CIRS patients that must be corrected. When you don't have adequate blood flow, cells begin to starve and cannot work properly.

VIP - Vasoactive Intestinal Polypeptide Normal Range: 23-63 pg/mL

Vasoactive intestinal polypeptide (VIP) is a neuro-regulatory hormone. VIP regulates cytokine responses, pulmonary artery pressures, and inflammation throughout the body.

Low VIP levels are present in CIRS patients (also in patients with multiple chemical sensitivity). This leads to unusual shortness of breath, especially in exercise. In the GI system, low VIP may cause watery diarrhea. VIP plays a role similar to MSH in regulating inflammatory responses.

VIP replacement, when used according to a strictly administered protocol, has proven to be extremely effective in returning chronically fatigued patients back to a normal life. **Do not start VIP if you are exposed to mold (with ERMI values greater than 2); if you fail a VCS test; or if you have MARCoNS present in your nose.** Serum lipase must be monitored as part of the VIP Protocol.

Lipase – Normal Range < 60 ug/ml

Lipase is an enzyme produced by the liver and pancreas to help digest fats. The lipase level in the blood is checked prior to the initiation of VIP nasal spray and again 30 days after VIP is started. Since VIP can raise lipase levels, patients are reminded to avoid supplements that contain lipase during VIP treatment.

GENOMIC TESTING

Recent advances in genomic science have given us a test known as **Progene DX**. This sophisticated blood test identifies proteins and/or genes that are differentially expressed in subjects suffering from CIRS, compared to healthy subjects. This lab test analyzes 50,000 genes to detect alterations in gene transcription. With this information, we now have new insights into not only CIRS, but also diseases like, Chronic Fatigue Syndrome, fibromyalgia, Post-Lyme Syndrome, and more. The test can be obtained on: www.survivingmold.com

---

NOTE: There have been arbitrary changes in the "Normal Reference Ranges" made by some labs, without explanation, in the past year. The reference ranges reflected in this document are the original values, used in the multiple clinical studies by Dr. Shoemaker and other Certified CIRS Practitioners.

In the Appendix, you will find the **Lab Results Tracking Form.** Use this form to keep track of your HLA-DR, Biomarkers, VCS, MARCoNS testing and ERMI/HERTSMI-2 testing as you progress through the protocol.

Laboratory Testing Challenges

Lab testing for specific biomarkers, in the Shoemaker Protocol, has not been an easy task for patients or practitioners. Several critically important lab tests have proven to be especially challenging. These include C4a, C3a, TGFb-1, MSH, MMP-9, VEGF, and VIP. These tests are essential for accurate diagnosis, tracking, and disease management.

Multiple facilities run these tests, using different methodologies and reference ranges. Only SPECIFIC LABS process specimens with the correct assay and exacting standars required for CIRS diagnosis and management. These are the ONLY labs, to date, that have produced consistently reliable and reproducible results on specific critical biomarkers.

Originally, Quest and LabCorp were the major carriers for most patients' insurance. Between the two facilities, these tests could be dispatched to the appropriate processing labs. However, there have been many recent changes.

Much effort is currently being made to streamline the process for obtaining accurate Biomarker Labs through Quest and LabCorp again. A potential comprehensive "Mold Panel", for all 7 biomarkers, is being evaluated by Quest.

NOTE: It is important to note that this information is subject to change at any point in time. It is the responsibility of the ordering practitioner, and designated office staff, to be aware of the most current laboratory requirements for accuracy. A few of the Certified CIRS Practitioners have private arrangements with the approved labs and can draw blood in their offices to be processed correctly. **Check the MOLD ILLNESS Facebook Page for ongoing updates.**

MSH- Must be run by LabCorp **only** through their Burlington, NC facility.

C4a/C3a- (Not Futhan) Must be run by **National Jewish** labs. Some third party and hospital labs do have contracts with National Jewish, but this will need to be verified in advance.

TGFB-1- **Cambridge Biomedical** is the preferred processor. Quest, and some 3rd party facilities, will send to Cambridge, but that needs to be guaranteed prior to specimen collection. LabCorp will not send to Cambridge, but will send to Viracor, which is acceptable.

MMP9- Must be run by **Esoterix**, a LabCorp company. Third party and hospital labs have been able to collect and send to either Labcorp or directly to Esoterix. Verification is necessary. **NOTE:** The "normal" reference range on the LabCorp site was recently changed and is NOT discriminating enough for CIRS tracking and management. The original reference range of 85-332 ng/ml is still used for CIRS.

VEGF- The correct assay is performed by Quest with an appropriate reference range.

VIP- This test is performed by **Quest** not by LabCorp. There have been some changes in the reference ranges that do not reflect individual values below 50, as they have in the past. Most CIRS patients are below the 50 range, and reporting of absolute values is important for tracking.

HLA DR- Can be done through **LabCorp or Quest**. Lab Corp uses only one code while Quest needs two run codes (15485 & 19526) to complete the HLA, DRB, and DQ categories. Low resolution testing is acceptable. Other labs, such as Life Extension, also offer HLA-DR testing.

Test codes are currently correct on the Physician Order Sheet on Survivingmold.com for:

1. HLA-DR to LabCorp
2. MSH to LabCorp
3. MMP9 to LabCorp
4. VEGF to Quest

When getting these labs drawn, it is helpful to have your doctor send in the order ahead of time. Then, schedule an appointment so that the lab can have the time to prepare for the collection. Often, the lab must take time to look up the collection requirements for labs that are not routinely done. This helps to expedite the process for everyone involved.

NOTE: These specialty lab tests can be expensive. IF your health insurance does NOT cover them, be sure to ask your lab about a CASH price. This can save you a significant amount of money.

Remember, you will be spending significant time in the lab each time you go. It is important to determine that the building is SAFE (has not had a history of water damage.) You do not want your medical experience to contribute to your exposure and worsen your condition!

Buildings like labs, drawing stations, and medical offices require the same careful scrutiny as other indoor environments that you visit...NO EXCEPTIONS!

History and Physical Exam:

A thorough history and physical exam are essential. Subtle signs and symptoms of CIRS can be accurately identified by an experienced CIRS Specialist. Elements of the physical exam are detailed in the Primary Care Practitioners' Overview in the Appendix.

Testing and Treatment of MARCoNS

MARCoNS stands for Multiply Antibiotic Resistant Coagulase Negative Staphylococcus. It lives in the deep nasal passages of the majority of people with CIRS. These bacteria form a sticky biofilm and release biotoxins. The biofilm coats and protects the bacteria from attack by the immune system or by antibiotics. The biotoxins depress MSH, a potent natural anti-inflammatory hormone. MARCoNS also has the potential to suppress C4a levels.

MARCoNS is diagnosed by a deep nasal swab, which is sent to Microbiology DX labs in Massachusetts. If it is present, and there are **at least 2 classes of antibiotic resistance**, treatment with a unique high potency colloidal silver nasal spray is used. 25 ppm of premium colloidal silver is compounded with EDTA and a special muco-adhesive polymer, to improve effectiveness. (Earlier versions of the protocol involved using BEG nasal spray and Rifampin, but use of those drugs is no longer recommended.)

(See Appendix for EDTA/Colloidal Silver/Mucolox Nasal Spray Instructions.)

Brain MRI with NeuroQuant (NQ):

A brain MRI, done without contrast, is used to identify characteristic brain changes that occur with CIRS. The NeuroQuant (NQ) is a computer program used to analyze the MRI images, after the test is completed. This program measures the volume of specific brain structures and can identify the unique "fingerprint" of CIRS on the brain. Specific machine settings need to be utilized on the MRI machine, in order to process the NQ. Your Certified Practitioner will need to write the order for your brain MRI with that specific information.

WHY DID I GET SICK?

Approximately 25% of the population is susceptible to CIRS. If you do NOT have a specific genetic profile, you are unlikely to be affected, even if you are exposed to the offending molds or mold by-products. This has led to many individuals CIRS being labeled as "crazy" when they proclaim that a particular environment is making them sick. Most others will be able to tolerate the same environment with no symptoms whatsoever!

The screening test for the genetic susceptibility to CIRS is known as the HLA-DR by PCR. This is a simple blood test that identifies the genetic profile you inherited. Human Leukocyte Antigens (HLAs) are found on the surface of nearly every cell in the human body. Their purpose is to help the immune system distinguish between "friend and foe", between "self" and "non-self."

The immune response genes are found on chromosome six. Everyone has two alleles for each gene. One is inherited from each biological parent. Based on Dr. Shoemaker's data, we know the frequency of mold illness-susceptible patients is approximately 25% of the general population. Almost a quarter of the normal population is genetically susceptible to chronic mold illness. The other three quarters is not.

To further complicate the picture, not everyone with the susceptible genetic profile will be ill. Those individuals who have clinical CIRS have

1. Experienced "activation" of their genetic blueprint and
2. Been exposed to the offending biotoxin (usually in a WDB)

It has been said that genetics 'loads the gun" and environmental exposure "pulls the trigger."

We are born with our genetic "blueprint", but the science of genomics has proven that specific genes may be expressed or repressed by environmental factors. An event that stresses our internal biochemistry may cause the immune system to go awry. Severe stress, illness, surgery, significant biotoxin exposure, high fever, pregnancy, etc. may trigger a cytokine storm and "activate" a CIRS susceptibility that was present from birth. **That means that the symptoms may begin at any age and lack of symptoms does not mean that you are immune to CIRS!**

WHAT ARE BIOTOXINS?

Biotoxins are produced by living organisms and can be found in (1) water damaged buildings, (2) ticks and brown recluse spiders, (3) blue-green algae (cyanobacteria), and (4) tropical fish contaminated by dinoflagellates such as Pfiesteria or Ciguatera.

80% of CIRS patients are ill because of their exposure to WDB.

Now let's look at exactly what is happening in CIRS. The Biotoxin Pathway outlines the evolution of the problem, step by step.

BIOTOXIN PATHWAY

Stage 1: Biotoxin Effects:

It all starts when a person is exposed to a biotoxin. In most people, the biotoxin is 'tagged' and identified by the body's immune system and is then broken down and removed from the blood by the liver. However, some individuals do not have the immune response genes (HLA-DR genes) that are required to form an antibody to a specific foreign antigen. In these cases, the biotoxins remain in the body indefinitely, free to circulate and cause massive inflammation.

Biotoxins also directly affect nerve cell function. This is why specific symptoms and the visual contrast sensitivity (VCS) test are so useful for diagnosis and for detecting re-exposure.

Stage 2: Cytokine Effects:

Cytokines (inflammatory proteins in the blood) bind to receptors on the cells, causing release of MMP9 in blood. In the brain, cytokines bind to the leptin receptor, preventing its normal function and reducing the production of MSH. Elevated cytokines can produce many different symptoms including: headache, muscle ache, unstable temperature and difficulty concentrating. This problem is the disastrous effect of MSH deficiency.

High levels of cytokines can also result in abnormal levels of clotting

factors. MMP-9 delivers inflammatory elements from the blood into sensitive tissues and can increase clot formation and blockage of circulation.

Stage 3: Reduced VEGF:

The elevated cytokine levels in the capillaries attract white blood cells, leading to restricted blood flow and lower oxygen levels in the tissues. Reduced VEGF leads to fatigue, muscle cramps, reduced exercise tolerance, and shortness of breath.

Stage 4: Immune System Effects:

Patients with certain HLA genotypes (immunity related genes) may develop inappropriate immune responses. These may include gluten sensitivity, autoimmune issues and blood clotting abnormalities. Most importantly, the complement system becomes chronically activated resulting in high levels of C4a. This reflects the "out of control" inflammation affecting virtually every system of the body, including the brain. Elevated levels of cytokines, like MMP-9, TGFB-1, and decreased MSH, can cause "leaky junctions" in both the gut and the blood brain barrier. This allows neuropathic toxins to enter the brain, resulting in widespread brain inflammation and dysregulation of the hypothalamus and pituitary.

Stage 5: Low MSH:

MSH is a hormone that controls other hormones, inflammation and immune system function. MSH is low in 95% of individuals with CIRS. When it is low, BAD things happen! Reduced MSH decreases the production of melatonin, which results in non-restorative sleep and chronic fatigue. Endorphin production is suppressed which leads to chronic and debilitating pain. Lack of MSH can cause mal-absorption or 'leaky gut'. This condition further weakens and deregulates the immune system. White blood cells eventually lose normal cytokine response so that opportunistic infections may occur and recovery from infection is slower.

Stage 6: Antibiotic Resistant Staph Bacteria

Reduced MSH also allows antibiotic-resistant staph bacteria (MARCoNS) to survive in biofilm on the mucous membranes. These bacteria further compound MSH deficiency by producing toxins that destroy MSH. At this point, the downward spiral starts to perpetuate itself.

Stage 7: Pituitary Hormone Effects

Reduced MSH can decrease pituitary production of antidiuretic hormone (ADH). This can lead to thirst, frequent urination, low blood pressure (especially on standing), low blood volume, and electric shocks from static electricity. While sex hormone production is often down-regulated the pituitary may up-regulate the production of cortisol and ACTH in the early stages of illness. These levels then drop to abnormally low, or low-normal ranges later as the illness progresses.

Adapted from: Dr. Ritchie Shoemaker, **www.survivingmold.com**

The Biotoxin Pathway

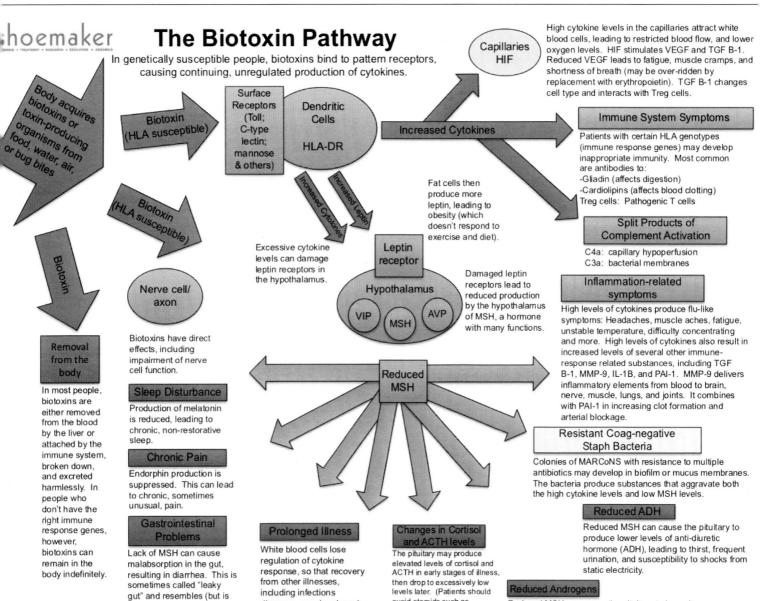

shoemaker

In genetically susceptible people, biotoxins bind to pattern receptors, causing continuing, unregulated production of cytokines.

Body acquires biotoxins or toxin-producing organisms from food, water, air, or bug bites

Biotoxin (HLA susceptible)

Biotoxin (HLA susceptible)

Biotoxin

Surface Receptors (Toll; C-type lectin; mannose & others)

Dendritic Cells

HLA-DR

Increased Cytokines

Increased Cytokines

Increased Leptin

Capillaries HIF

High cytokine levels in the capillaries attract white blood cells, leading to restricted blood flow, and lower oxygen levels. HIF stimulates VEGF and TGF B-1. Reduced VEGF leads to fatigue, muscle cramps, and shortness of breath (may be over-ridden by replacement with erythropoietin). TGF B-1 changes cell type and interacts with Treg cells.

Immune System Symptoms

Patients with certain HLA genotypes (immune response genes) may develop inappropriate immunity. Most common are antibodies to:
-Gliadin (affects digestion)
-Cardiolipins (affects blood clotting)
Treg cells: Pathogenic T cells

Fat cells then produce more leptin, leading to obesity (which doesn't respond to exercise and diet).

Excessive cytokine levels can damage leptin receptors in the hypothalamus.

Leptin receptor

Damaged leptin receptors lead to reduced production by the hypothalamus of MSH, a hormone with many functions.

Hypothalamus

VIP   **MSH**   **AVP**

Split Products of Complement Activation

C4a: capillary hypoperfusion
C3a: bacterial membranes

Inflammation-related symptoms

High levels of cytokines produce flu-like symptoms: Headaches, muscle aches, fatigue, unstable temperature, difficulty concentrating and more. High levels of cytokines also result in increased levels of several other immune-response related substances, including TGF B-1, MMP-9, IL-1B, and PAI-1. MMP-9 delivers inflammatory elements from blood to brain, nerve, muscle, lungs, and joints. It combines with PAI-1 in increasing clot formation and arterial blockage.

Nerve cell/ axon

Biotoxins have direct effects, including impairment of nerve cell function.

Reduced MSH

Removal from the body

In most people, biotoxins are either removed from the blood by the liver or attached by the immune system, broken down, and excreted harmlessly. In people who don't have the right immune response genes, however, biotoxins can remain in the body indefinitely.

Sleep Disturbance

Production of melatonin is reduced, leading to chronic, non-restorative sleep.

Chronic Pain

Endorphin production is suppressed. This can lead to chronic, sometimes unusual, pain.

Gastrointestinal Problems

Lack of MSH can cause malabsorption in the gut, resulting in diarrhea. This is sometimes called "leaky gut" and resembles (but is not) celiac disease. IBS is often present.

Prolonged Illness

White blood cells lose regulation of cytokine response, so that recovery from other illnesses, including infections diseases, may be slowed.

Changes in Cortisol and ACTH levels

The pituitary may produce elevated levels of cortisol and ACTH in early stages of illness, then drop to excessively low levels later. (Patients should avoid steroids such as prednisone, which can lower levels of ACTH)

Resistant Coag-negative Staph Bacteria

Colonies of MARCoNS with resistance to multiple antibiotics may develop in biofilm or mucus membranes. The bacteria produce substances that aggravate both the high cytokine levels and low MSH levels.

Reduced ADH

Reduced MSH can cause the pituitary to produce lower levels of anti-diuretic hormone (ADH), leading to thirst, frequent urination, and susceptibility to shocks from static electricity.

Reduced Androgens

Reduced MSH can cause the pituitary to lower its production of sex hormones.

©R. Shoemaker, 2011

STEP BY STEP ACTION PLAN

1. **Making a definitive diagnosis** is the first step on your road to recovery. Diagnosis begins with a detailed and comprehensive history and physical exam. Specific diagnostic tests for CIRS are collected and reviewed.

2. **Use appropriate Environmental Testing:** ERMI/HERTSMI-2 testing is done to detect the current level of specific biotoxins. Building performance is also evaluated. Additional techniques might be indicated in specific situations.

3. **Remove from biotoxin exposure**, whether at home, work, school or other venue. **If exposure is ongoing, the protocol will NOT work.** Cross contamination exposure must also be carefully evaluated.

4. **Correct toxin levels in the body with CSM** (Cholestyramine) or Welchol, using VCS testing to monitor progress. These drugs bind toxins so they can be eliminated. The visual contrast test confirms resolving inflammation as the toxin levels drop.

5. **Eradicate biofilm-forming MARCoNS.** These bacteria promote continued inflammation, immune dysfunction, and low MSH. Once they are eliminated with EDTA/Colloidal Silver/Mucolox Nasal Spray, your immune system is able to respond appropriately to the remaining steps of the protocol.

6. **Eliminate gluten** for those with anti-gliadin antibodies. Avoiding gluten allows the antibody levels to fall so inflammation will improve.

7. **Correct elevated MMP-9** (Matrix Metallopeptidase-9) levels. This enzyme causes "leaky" blood vessels and allows inflammatory chemicals to enter the muscle, nerve, brain and joint tissues. This causes severe pain and inflammation.

High dose fish oils and a low amylose diet will help to reduce MMP-9 and improve symptoms of headache, muscle and joint pain and stiffness.

8. **Correct ADH** (anti-diuretic hormone). A low ADH often causes dehydration, thirst, frequent urination, headaches and static "shocks." DDAVP nasal spray (or tablet) restores your body's ability to hold on to water appropriately and relieves these symptoms.

9. **Correct low VEGF** (Vascular Endothelial Growth Factor). This protein stimulates the growth of blood vessels and dilates blood vessels to improve blood flow and oxygen delivery to the tissues. In CIRS, VEGF is low, so there is no way to increase blood flow during exercise. Persistent fatigue, muscle aches and cognitive problems can result. High dose fish oil helps to restore VEGF.

10. **Correct elevated C3a**, due to the presence of bacteria, often seen in Lyme disease. When this persists, after appropriate antibiotic treatment, it is treated with high dose statin drugs, for a limited time. CoQ10 is used to combat side effects of the statins.

11. **Correct elevated C4a**, due to the diffuse inflammation caused by CIRS-WDB. C4a levels will fall as the patient responds to the earlier steps of the protocol. If C4a remains persistently elevated, it will be corrected by VIP at the end of the protocol.

12. **Reduce elevated TGF beta-1** (Transforming Growth Factor). This protein causes dysfunctional changes in tissues, lowers VEGF, and stimulates auto-immune issues. TGFB-1 generally falls as inflammation resolves. If it remains elevated, it can be treated at this point with losartan. Blood pressure monitoring is important during the 30 day therapy, as losartan will reduce blood pressure.

13. **Optimize VIP** (Vasoactive Intestinal Peptide) if the patient is still symptomatic after completing each of the above steps. VIP has the ability to not only correct the important biomarker abnormalities, but to restore the regulation of the innate immune system. Specific criteria must be met prior to beginning VIP and lipase levels must be monitored. (See Appendix for instructions.)

14. **Final check to verify stability off meds.** A check of biomarkers, VCS, and symptom inventory is done at the conclusion of therapy. A Progene CIRS assay

re-test and MRI with Neuro-Quant will also provide valuable information on the clinical status. Ongoing diligence and symptom tracking is essential. Any suspected re-exposure needs to be promptly evaluated and treated appropriately.

Once patients have completed the protocol, we advise keeping CSM on hand to use preventatively if they will be entering a "questionable" environment. It is also a good idea to use the CSM for a few days if symptoms and VCS suggest a re-exposure.

NOTE: A detailed version of the Shoemaker Protocol can be found in the Appendix - **Shoemaker Protocol: Guidelines for Primary Care Providers.**

TRACKING DAILY ACTIVITY

AN ESSENTIAL SURVIVAL SKILL

Patient tracking is a systematic approach to identify your body's response to a specific action you have taken. It requires developing a daily awareness of the activities you are engaging in, and documenting this in a meaningful way. Tracking allows you to identify where the changes in your symptoms are coming from. Subtle changes in your symptoms may go undetected without diligent and systematic observation and documentation.

With this information, you have the ability to take control. You can decide to avoid the particular environment or activity that caused a negative physical response. Tracking can also help you to identify what actions and activities are helping you to improve.

One of the most critically important things to track, if you have been diagnosed with CIRS-WDB, are the environments you choose to enter. In this manual, we share many ways to recognize and avoid potentially contaminated buildings. With 50% of all buildings estimated to have water damage, it is essential to be selective about what buildings you choose to enter. **You will learn vital observation and documentation skills that will permit you to take charge of your situation, rather than being a victim of your diagnosis.**

If tracking is not incorporated into the treatment plan, critical pieces in the puzzle remain missing. This can lead the patient and the practitioner to attribute symptoms to causes that may not be responsible for the problem. This may cause further delays in treatment and recovery. Without tracking, patients will often be unaware of a building that is causing ongoing exposure.

Example: A patient's lab work was reviewed by a practitioner. It revealed elevated inflammatory markers as compared to the previous results. (The current lab work was done 3 weeks prior to the medical consult.) When the patient was asked if she remembered being exposed to a water damaged building prior to getting her labs drawn she replied, "No, I have not been to any other buildings during that time." During the interview with the practitioner, she continued to insist that she could not have been exposed during that time period. A few days after her consult, this patient remembered that she had spent a weekend at her mother's beach house during the time in question. This correlated with the elevation in her inflammatory markers and changes in her VCS testing.

This is a very common situation for CIRS patients and practitioners. **It would be difficult for most anyone to remember everywhere they have been, but for the CIRS patient it now becomes critical to their health and well-being.** It is also important to note that some common symptoms of CIRS can be brain fog, memory problems, and confusion. This makes the utilization of tracking even more important to help guide the treatment process.

Tracking for changes includes environments entered, any increase or decrease in symptoms, activity levels, starting or stopping any medications, supplements, treatments, therapies, or dietary recommendations. For example, starting massage therapy, acupuncture, or Epsom salt baths should be included in your tracking.

Any of these therapies can create a positive or negative response for a CIRS patient. A person so sick, and struggling for answers to help them feel better, will often engage in more of these activities than their body can tolerate. Certain treatments, supplements, and medications may work as intended for the person who is not affected by CIRS, but those same things may cause a negative reaction in a CIRS patient.

When the Biotoxin Pathway is activated in CIRS, massive systemic inflammation occurs. This inflammation, along with the increasing burden of toxins, severely impairs the body's ability to regulate, process, and excrete toxic substances. Until the patient is out of exposure, the body's total toxic burden reduced, and biomarkers corrected through use of the Shoemaker Protocol, conventional "cleansing" or "detox" therapies will put undue stress on the body.

Worsening of symptoms can come from many different situations or activities including: exposure to chemicals, preparations to "cleanse" or "detox" the body, supplements to stimulate increased immune function, or medications to kill bacteria, fungus, and viruses. Patients have even been confused about the source of their symptoms in the first 24 hours after being exposed to a cold or other virus. This is where VCS testing is so helpful, along with objective lab data, to determine mold exposure. Including tracking can help to pinpoint the offending activity almost immediately, without having to suffer needlessly for weeks.

It is easy to see that, without paying attention to the big picture of where you are going and what you are doing, it becomes impossible to control all the variables that exist for a CIRS patient. Without observing and systematically documenting the details, CIRS becomes a constantly fluctuating collection of symptoms, without any clear cause. This creates confusion and frustration for both the patient and the practitioner, as both search for the "WHY?".

When symptoms of CIRS develop in a patient, after an exposure, those symptoms will typically reappear in a predictable manner. This means that if you developed a scratchy throat or cough, headache, brain fog or a "spacey" feeling in your head after entering a building, it is important to make note of it. **If these symptoms are due to exposure, then the same group of symptoms will likely appear, if you are exposed to another moldy environment in the future.** When these symptoms occur within a few minutes of being in a new environment it is a signal for you to get out right away.

You will note that the symptoms listed above all involve the nose, throat, sinuses and brain. When you experience **immediate symptoms** (within just a few minutes of exposure) this generally means that the WDB is heavily contaminated and highly toxic. The biotoxins travel from the air, to your nose and sinuses, through the olfactory bulb and directly to the brain.

Sometimes a building will not produce immediate symptoms, but may cause them to occur hours later. A different group of reliable symptoms will typically be reproduced. Your specific and predictable delayed symptoms might include joint pain, muscle pain, muscle twitching, and fatigue. These are related to system-wide inflammation, once the biotoxins have entered the bloodstream and activated the innate immune system.

Example: You experience and document these reliable warning signs. You notice they are not connected to any activity you have done in the past 24-48 hours. However, with tracking your activity, you see that two days before, you spent 2 hours in a restaurant that had no obvious signs of water damage.

Tracking becomes a life skill a CIRS patient can't be without! Achieving success with the protocol, and recovering your health, depends on proactive observation and documentation. Fortunately, at the end of the Protocol, VIP can help with extreme reactivity. **However, avoidance of WDBs remains the number one lifelong priority!** Learning this can be inconvenient, and take time at first, but the benefits for the long term are immeasurable. With practice, it can become incorporated into your lifestyle.

Weekly tracking identifies common symptoms, buildings visited, medications, supplements, treatments, and any other significant events or changes. **Identifying what is affecting your health, and if the effect is negative, positive, or neutral, is critical and can be empowering and life altering.**

Example: This patient has had an early diagnosis of CIRS and obtained treatment from a practitioner. She finds that she just can't seem to make steady progress with her illness. She is now learning about tracking.

The patient lists five of her most troublesome symptoms with exposure. In her case, these are brain fog, muscle aches, joint pain, muscle twitching, and fatigue. It is confirmed that her home, grocery store, and church have been safe for her. She has been taking a whole food multivitamin, omega-3 fish oil, vitamin D, turmeric, and a probiotic. CSM is now used, at this point in her treatment, when she has an exposure. It is also used to help prevent symptoms of exposure when going into an unknown environment, if she remembers to take it beforehand.

Weekly tracking forms have room for additional symptoms that occur, buildings entered, treatments, and supplements/medications (*In Appendix*)

Day 1: There are no changes.

Day 2: The patient goes to a post office and a hardware store she had not been in before.

Day 3: She notices an increase in 2 common symptoms. She doesn't attribute them at this point to the buildings she was in. On this day, she needs to get something from a sealed container in the garage that has contaminated items from her old home. The patient also starts to take a glutathione spray and a liver supplement in hopes of making her feel better. They have worked great according to her friends and she has wanted to try them.

Day 4: The patient notices an increase in all 5 of her common symptoms plus headache and a burning in her sinuses. She stops the liver supplement.

Day 5: She is still experiencing close to the same level of increase in all 5 common symptoms, although one of her new symptoms is no longer there. Family members stop by this evening and after a few minutes of small talk she learns they are sick with colds! She stops the glutathione spray and starts CSM.

Day 6: She recognizes her 5 common symptoms and one new one are decreasing.

Day 7: She has returned to her previous state before the week's events and changes in her routine.

She is able to recognize, through tracking, several things she did that most likely contributed to her increase in symptoms.

There were six separate activities that this patient engaged in during the week that could have been responsible for her change in symptoms. This included 3 possible activities that lead to direct exposure to mold toxins, 2 activities where supplements she ingested can cause a possible negative systemic response, and one direct exposure to a possible virus or bacterial infection. Three of those activities she initiated on the same day! She had 14 changes in her symptoms in that week alone.

On day 2, looking back, she sees that she could have been exposed in one or both buildings she took a chance on entering without any kind of investigating beforehand. She forgot to take any CSM or Welchol, 2 hours before going into an unfamiliar building on day 2.

On day 3, she most likely experienced an exposure when opening a contaminated container without precautions. Not thinking about her recent activities and possible exposures, she tries 2 different supplements, at the same time, that can stimulate detoxification symptoms.

Day 4 is her worst day, but it is not known that any one or all the above could have elicited these responses. She stops one of the supplements she began on day three.

Day 5 she stops the other supplement started on day three not knowing if it is helping or making her feel worse. She is then exposed to a possible virus/ bacteria that could potentially create other symptoms for her over the next 24 to 48 hours confusing the picture even more.

She starts CSM as she figures out the activities that could have exposed her to biotoxins in the past week.

Day 6 she finds her symptoms subsiding.

Day 7 she is finally back to where she started (before she went about her week without thinking where she was going and what she was doing.)

This case is relatively simple in comparison with many others. **It provides a realistic picture of the many things that can happen in a single day to cause dramatic or subtle changes in symptoms for someone with CIRS.**

A WORD ON SUPPLEMENTS:

1. As you can see by the example above, supplements, just like medications, can have a powerful effect in initiating changes in the body. When your body's foundational operating systems are not functioning normally, a substance used to correct, stimulate or increase a process that is already struggling, may have negative consequences.

2. There are many helpful, high quality, scientifically validated supplements available for patients and practitioners. One must be cautious about using ANY substance, in CIRS, especially those that can impact the immune system or detox pathways. Even "natural" remedies can send a CIRS patient into a "tailspin"!

CIRS patients sometimes feel abandoned by traditional medicine practitioners and turn to natural alternatives for relief. These patients may take multiple supplements, with multiple actions, at one time. This creates confusion because the patient and practitioner are unable to determine which substance is making symptoms better or worse. Some of these supplements can worsen an underlying imbalance that already exists or overtax a fragile body chemistry.

People often ask about liver/gallbladder flushes. These can be helpful for certain patients. However, your practitioner will need to determine if this is appropriate for you and when would be the safest time for this to be utilized.

3. It is important to avoid treating symptoms, whether with medication or supplements, without treating the underlying cause. This common

mistake can lead the CIRS patient down a road that will add more problems than resolutions in the long term.

4. There is a right time and place to incorporate helpful formulas to assist the healing process, under the care and supervision of the CIRS practitioner. **Starting supplements at any time, in substitution of the Shoemaker Protocol, for a correctly diagnosed CIRS patient, will impede progress and prevent recovery.**

5. Supplements need to be carefully used and appropriately selected for each individual. **Only one new intervention at a time,** is the rule of thumb in CIRS. Staying consistent with an intervention, once started, is important while carefully observing for changes. Tracking responses to each intervention gives us the information needed to progress safely and effectively.

6. Supplements need to be routinely evaluated for proper dosage, effect, and need, based on patient tracking and appropriate lab monitoring.

CIRS is a master at mimicking other diseases. Treating what may appear to be multiple illnesses, without clearly understanding the multi-system symptoms of CIRS, is a common mistake.

If CIRS is suspected, a definitive diagnosis is obtained by a CIRS Certified Practitioner, using specific objective parameters. Protocols are followed precisely, and many of the symptoms, thought to be caused by another disease state, will resolve by following the protocols and correcting underlying imbalances.

Example:
A classic example of "over-reach" in a CIRS patient is a 48 year old female with diagnosed CIRS. She failed her VCS test, had a susceptible HLA-DR, and demonstrated 21 symptoms of CIRS. Her biomarkers were predictably elevated and her ERMI was extremely high.

While her home is being remediated by a CIRS literate mold specialist, she begins Cholestyramine to bind the biotoxins, under the direction of her CIRS Certified Practitioner. She continues to complain of severe skin itching and "crawling" sensations under her skin. She is scratching, rubbing, and "picking" at her skin almost constantly. She has researched online and is convinced that she has Morgellons Disease. Her primary care provider did a skin biopsy, which was negative. She was referred for a mental health evaluation.

Symptoms of CIRS include unusual skin sensations such as itching, burning, tingling, prickling, and crawling sensations. These are common and NOT likely due to a secondary cause. Once the binders removed the biotoxins, and the innate immune system had a chance to recover, systemic inflammation resolved and her skin symptoms disappeared.

In discussing this situation with a friend who is a naturopathic physician, he replied, "Now I 'get it.' The natural therapies and supplements I use are kinder and gentler than most pharmaceuticals. Still, if the body systems are not capable of responding appropriately, trying to enhance detoxification or support immunity, can make the situation worse! Asking the body to perform functions it is not currently capable of, merely adds more stress and dysfunction." EXACTLY!

The message is to keep your eye on the ball! Critical and sequential thinking is essential. Once the diagnosis of CIRS is made, using the appropriate objective criteria, use the Shoemaker Protocol PRECISELY. Keep other interventions to a minimum until underlying dysregulation of multiple body systems is corrected.

NOTE: Tracking forms for symptoms are found in the Appendix. (More details on tracking a little later.) We will also present specific & simple tools to use prior to entering a building. Helpful acronyms for mold exposure prevention, and "scripts" for communicating your specific needs, related to CIRS, will make your day-to-day life much easier to manage.

EXERCISE AND CIRS

CIRS patients notice an inability to perform meaningful exercise to sustain any degree of muscle strength or fitness. Fatigue is a very common symptom. Well-meaning friends and professionals will often recommend incorporating an exercise program to help combat this. Those who are not familiar with CIRS do not understand the ongoing effects of inflammation in the body of a patient. An exercise program, prior to initiating the Shoemaker Protocol, will not benefit the patient and can often make things worse. Here is why.

Decreased VEGF (vascular endothelial growth factor) results from high levels of cytokines in capillaries. This attracts white blood cells which leads to restricted blood flow (hypo-perfusion) and low levels of oxygen in the tissues. This leads to fatigue, muscle cramps, and shortness of breath, as explained in the Biotoxin Pathway basics.

For some patients, walking up a small flight of stairs can leave them completely out of breath. Others may notice a more gradual decline in their endurance and ability to exercise over time, despite their best efforts. Even when a patient is progressing, too much strenuous activity can make recovery more difficult. It is important to know that capillary hypo-perfusion reduces the amount of blood and oxygen available to the muscles. When there is reduced oxygen delivery, muscles quickly starve. When this happens, the body converts to using anaerobic energy systems that don't require oxygen.

When anaerobic energy systems produce a buildup of lactic acid, faster than it can be cleared away, this is called "exceeding the anaerobic threshold." When this happens, there is also a breakdown of protein to be used for fuel. Glycogen stores in the muscles, normally used as a secondary source for long term energy, are also used inefficiently.

What does this mean for the CIRS patient? Avoiding exercise that exceeds the anaerobic threshold is very important. Exercise must be gradually introduced at the proper time, slowly and methodically. **Those individuals who attempt to do too much, too quickly, will experience the "PUSH and CRASH" effect. Feeling good one day, and exerting yourself beyond your usual capacity, will result in exhaustion and muscle soreness, often for several days!**

Your CIRS Certified Practitioner can guide you in an exercise "prescription" to meet your individual needs, when the time is appropriate. The general guidelines include:

1. Exercise is to be done DAILY....no exceptions.
2. Start with 5 minutes of walking or exercise bike with NO incline or resistance.
3. If tolerated well, add 2 minutes to the exercise time daily until you can tolerate 15 minutes. *(Nothing is gained beyond 15 min.)*
4. Next, after 15 min. of treadmill or bike, add 5 minutes of abdominal exercises *(on the floor – sit-ups, leg lifts, crunches).*
5. If tolerated well, add 2 minutes daily to abdominal routine until at 15 min. *(no more than 15 min. is recommended.)*
6. Finally, after 15 min. cardio and 15 min. abdominal exercises are accomplished, without experiencing unusual fatigue or muscle pain, add upper body workout *(biceps, triceps, pecs, etc.)* with 2.5 lb. weights. Start with 8 reps for each muscle group and increase gradually to a total of 15 minutes for this routine as well.

Now your total daily exercise routine is at 45 minutes. At this point, you can begin to gradually add resistance to the bike, slight incline to the abdominal workout, and small increments of weight to the upper body routine. This needs to be done one at a time and gradually.

These exercise recommendations are not arbitrary. DAILY incremental increases in exercise will increase a substance known as adiponectin, a hormone that regulates fat metabolism. This hormone allows you to burn fatty acids much more effectively and dramatically increases the energy available to your muscles. Within two to three months, you will see a dramatic improvement in exercise tolerance. Skipping a day of exercise will slow your progress significantly.

Lactic acid build up in the muscles is painful and depleting the body's fuel reserves can contribute to debilitating and long lasting fatigue. **Similar symptoms can also be caused by exposure to toxins. It is critically important to be aware of where symptoms are coming from in CIRS.** This can be extremely confusing if a patient is not tracking the changes in their activities, as well as their potential exposures. Physical activity is an essential category to document on your tracking form. *(See Appendix)*

THE EMOTIONAL TOLL OF CIRS

The individual with CIRS faces a number of unique challenges:

The illness affects nearly every body system, producing a wide variety of seemingly unrelated symptoms, which are often constant and unremitting.

Because CIRS is confined almost exclusively to individuals with a specific activated genetic blueprint, other family, friends & co-workers who are in the same environment may remain symptom free.

While a few specific tests can conclusively establish the diagnosis, these are NOT tests that are widely used in medical offices. Common screening laboratory tests are usually normal and offer no clues to CIRS.

The biochemical reactions and widespread "out of control" inflammation may cause incapacitating fatigue and pain while the individual may not, at least initially, "look sick."

At this time, the number of Certified CIRS Practitioners is limited. Fortunately, that number is growing steadily. The medical community at large is just becoming aware of CIRS. If the disease is not "on the radar" for your practitioner, it will not even be considered as a possibility in establishing your diagnosis.

Because "brain-fog", sleep disturbance, memory loss and mood disorders are often caused by the rampant inflammation of CIRS, many patients are told they are anxious, depressed, bipolar, or simply that the illness is "all in their head." Many have been misdiagnosed with fibromyalgia, chronic fatigue syndrome, MS, Alzheimer's disease and others.

Because the biotoxin burden is cumulative, and the CIRS individual is unable to process and remove these toxins, the disease will follow a downward spiral until effective treatment is begun.

As if the above issues are not difficult enough, the CIRS is usually being caused by the patient's home environment. Exhaustive testing is then followed by a difficult decision to invest in a thorough and painstaking remediation or move to a new "safe" environment. As the patient becomes increasingly ill, he or she spends more time at home. That means more time in the very environment that is probably contributing most to the illness.

It is easy to see why individuals with CIRS are often discouraged, angry, depressed, or suffer from low self-esteem. Relationships suffer as family members feel frustrated and powerless. This disease takes a toll on the entire family.

CIRS is REAL!

CIRS is not difficult to diagnose with the appropriate evaluation, by a qualified CIRS practitioner.

Most importantly, CIRS can be effectively treated, and patients and families can reclaim their lives. It happens every day.

It is time for individuals with CIRS to be seen, heard, recognized, and treated appropriately, with a scientifically validated treatment protocol that WORKS!

NOTE: In the Appendix, you will find **"Facts about CIRS for Friends & Family."**

This handout can be copied and given to the people in your life who need to understand what CIRS is and how it affects you.

There are also sample letter templates for your employer, school, and landlord/seller. Your CIRS Certified Practitioner can personalize these for you on their professional letterhead. These letters will lend support for your unique medical needs in specific situations.

DO I NEED A CERTIFIED CIRS PRACTITIONER?

CIRS is an extremely complex illness, still very new to the medical community. While more doctors and nurse practitioners are learning about CIRS every day, few have the in depth knowledge to accurately diagnose and treat this illness with long-term success. Many practitioners will "cherry-pick", using bits and pieces of the protocol to see what results might be achieved. **You deserve the benefit of hard science and what has been PROVEN in more than 10,000 patients, not just someone's "best guess."**

I love my family practitioner, but I would not rely upon him to do a knee replacement or heart surgery. There are times that only a specialist, with a unique understanding and skill set, will be able to help you achieve the best results. **This often misunderstood illness must be managed by a knowledgeable team of specialists who are diligent and relentless in practicing the highest standard of care for CIRS patients.**

NOTE: You can obtain a list of currently Certified CIRS Practitioners at www.survivingmold.com

---

WHAT DOES MY PRIMARY CARE PRACTITIONER NEED TO KNOW?

Your primary care provider has the important role of coordinating your health care. He or she will likely be able to manage your ongoing monitoring after you have completed the Shoemaker Protocol with a Certified CIRS Practitioner.

An Overview of the Shoemaker Protocol for Primary Care Practitioners has been provided in the Appendix. This is a more detailed medical version of the **Step by Step** document. We suggest that you copy this document for your Primary Care Provider to read and then file in your chart. This information will provide a larger perspective from which to manage your comprehensive health needs.

HOW DO I KNOW IF A BUILDING IS WATER DAMAGED?

Most people assume that a water damaged building (WDB) will always smell moldy, look moldy, and have deteriorated building materials that indicate some degree of "moldiness". While some buildings do have obvious examples of moldiness, many do not. A water event is likely to happen sometime during a buildings life cycle. In fact, environmental experts estimate that 50% of buildings in the U.S. currently have water damage significant enough to impact an individual with CIRS.

It's important to understand the level of contamination that can occur when a water event happens. The Institute of Inspection, Cleaning and Restoration Certification (IIRC) categorizes water intrusion and damage according to the source of the water. Although all water poses potential health problems, there are levels of risk depending on the event as detailed below:

Category 1: Clean water originates from a source that does not immediately pose substantial harm to humans. This includes broken water supply lines, tub or sink overflows with no contaminates, appliance malfunctions involving water supply lines, melting snow or ice, and falling rain water.

Category 2: "Grey water" carries a significant level of contamination. It has the potential to cause illness to humans. Grey water sources may include discharge from dishwashers or washing machines, over flow from toilets with some urine no feces, and seepage due to hydrostatic pressure (i.e. concrete slab leak).

Category 3: "Black water" contains disease-causing agents and is grossly unsanitary. Sewage backflow that originates from beyond the toilet trap is considered black water contamination, regardless of visible content or color.

The levels of risk between a category one water damage and a category three can be vastly different in how it affects the "general population**." In an individual with a "gene activated" CIRS, a category one event that causes even a "little bit" of water damage, can be just as influential in causing CIRS symptoms as a category two or three event.**

Mold symptoms are not "dose dependent". This means that even small amounts of exposure can trigger the immune system to start the damaging cascade of inflammation. The severity of the symptoms will depend on the toxicity of the building combined with the current state of illness for the CIRS individual. Those who have had CIRS for a longer period of time, and been re-exposed on multiple occasions, will likely experience the "sicker quicker" phenomenon. More severe and diffuse symptoms will occur with less and less exposure.

This is why, even if you are living in a healthy environment and go to a grocery store that has had water damage, you may find that even a few minutes of exposure can put you back in bed, re-living your symptoms for days. **This also emphasizes the importance of asking your doctor, dentist, therapist, lab, etc. if their buildings have had any water damage. Certainly, any CIRS Medical Provider should have their office ERMI tested for safety.**

Toxins are the root cause. It is critical to understand that old water damage, as well as recent water damage, can be toxic to the CIRS individual. It only takes 48 hours for mold growth to occur after a water intrusion, given the right conditions. Toxins from mold spores are not alive or dead. Historic water damage, that has long since been "remediated", may still have toxins present if proper removal of all toxins has not taken place. It is critical that no toxins remain.

It is vital to understand that the contents within a water-damaged building are considered contaminated until tested and proven otherwise. This applies even if the contents are located in another part of the building that was not directly exposed to the water intrusion. The mold, mold fragments, bacteria, toxins, and

inflammatory chemicals are invisible and travel through the air, infiltrating every nook and cranny of a WDB.

CIRS individuals cannot expect to continue to expose themselves to toxins. This awareness and understanding is critical to their successful treatment and overall quality of life. Many CIRS individuals will come to learn that they will get "sick quicker" as they continue to either live in a toxic environment or find themselves getting repeatedly re-exposed by entering a toxic environment.

WHERE DO I START WHEN MY HOME MAY BE THE PROBLEM?

Finding environmental professionals with a complete understanding of what CIRS individuals require, and how to make that happen in the most practical way possible, has been a daunting task.

There is a limited current resource list in the appendix. New resources will become available over time. These can be accessed by going to: www.survivingmold.com. This illness may require multiple resources to support and defend CIRS individuals from emotional and financial ruin as they try to make sense of their illness, and seek qualified help in the process.

To help the CIRS individual choose potential resources, there are checklists within the appendix. These checklists are to be used as a guide to educate the individual and help to select CIRS literate, qualified professionals. These are NOT to be used as "Do It Yourself" instructions.

ENVIRONMENTAL ASSESSMENT

The CIRS treatment protocol requires that CIRS individuals remove themselves from toxin exposure. The choice to move or stay is dependent on several factors and needs to be based upon thorough and specific evaluation. Your Indoor Environmental Professional (IEP) should be responsible for assessing your environment (i.e. home, school, work place) and creating a personalized work plan that may include remediation, building, cleaning, content cleaning, building back with the right materials to minimize future water damage, and using building science to prevent cross contamination within the building.

Much like your Surviving Mold (SM) certified health care professional, an IEP who has direct experience with correcting buildings for the CIRS individual, is a critical part of your health care team. The IEP and the SM Certified Practitioner should be in direct communication and have clear open exchange of information to support the success of the patient. There are currently very few IEP's who have direct field experience with CIRS individuals. For this reason, we have provided an assessment checklist specific to evaluating environments for a CIRS individual. (See Appendix)

This assessment checklist can also be used as a guide to assist you when soliciting the services of an IEP and others. The checklist will help educate and create awareness for the service providers of specific points that might be overlooked in a "standard" building assessment. Awareness of specific details can save time, money, and frustration when you are talking about creating an environment that will be safe for CIRS occupancy. (See assessment check list in the Appendix.)

In addition to the assessment checklist, we recommend filling out the "Initial Intake form" located in the Appendix. Complete this form and submit it to your CIRS health care professional as well as the IEP. This tool will provide them with a good starting point regarding your health history as well as the history detailing water events that have occurred in your home. Often, while completing this form, the CIRS patient, health care professional, and IEP, can identify relevant exposure sources and begin to understand the link between the CIRS individual's symptoms and events in their life (i.e. water damage, traumatic events). For many, it is truly a revelation when these links and correlations are made.

Remember, your exposure can be from old water damage that you were not aware of, or from exposed contents that you brought with you. Household contents may contaminate each new environment as you re-locate those items. It is also possible for family members to bring mold toxins home from their work or school environment. There can be many different sources of exposure.

The more information you can reveal to your IEP and health care professional, the more thorough the investigation will be. The initial intake form, in combination with the environmental assessment, helps to identify environmental problems and their correlation with symptoms more accurately. Having clear information can be life changing! Most CIRS individuals, up to this point in their illness, may have a diagnosis, but no clear path forward. By collecting very specific and critical details, your IEP and your medical practitioner will have the necessary information to help you chart your path to recovery.

How much exposure is SAFE?

An important way to know that you are in a "safe" environment is to monitor your biomarkers, physical symptoms, and VCS testing on a regular basis. While some individuals are able to feel when they have been exposed within minutes of the exposure, others may not have symptoms until hours or days later. Ongoing exposure to a "less sick" building, where symptoms for the patient may be less obvious, will still be harmful, over time, for the CIRS patient.

For those who are extremely ill, symptom changes from a re-exposure can seem non-existent or very subtle. These individuals feel so ill on a regular basis, it is difficult for them to detect when new or increasing symptoms occur. These patients will share that they feel "bad" all the time and sometimes they feel even worse. After starting the treatment program for CIRS, patients have more ability to notice when these changes happen.

They feel better and are able to recognize when a certain set of symptoms occurs after being exposed. **Early detection of subtle or significant changes in physical symptoms, with the help of tracking, allows the patient to avoid unsafe exposure.**

The noninvasive visual contrast sensitivity test (VCS) is an effective way to monitor how different environments may be affecting you, without waiting weeks for test results. Exposures will change the results of this test for the majority of people within 24 – 36 hours. It is a very valuable tool for both patients and practitioners. It can be performed online for a nominal fee. See: **www.survivingmold.com**.

HOW DO I EFFECTIVELY TEST FOR MOLD?

Testing for mold for a CIRS individual is very different than testing for mold for the rest of the population. For a CIRS individual, in addition to the current mold condition of the environment, the historical mold data must be known. Once again, it is the toxin that is affecting the health of the CIRS individual, and the toxin is not a live or dead entity. For example, old water damage may have produced mold related toxins decades ago. These toxins may still be present and therefore be the source of the problem.

As for the various methods of testing for mold, the most critical difference is that out of fifteen different methods of testing commonly used, only one test can give all of the results shown below by using the scientific technology of the **MSQPCR (mold-specific quantitative polymerase chain reaction) method.**

- SPECIES
- SPORE VIABILITY
- SPORE FRAGMENTS
- HYPHAE
- HYPHAL FRAGMENTS
- HEALTH/SAFETY EXPOSURE

This test is known as Environmental Relative Moldiness Index or ERMI. It must be performed by qualified licensed lab such as Mycometrics. (See Resources) The health care practitioner can use the results to evaluate the health effects for the patient by using what is called the HERTSMI-2 scoring method. (Health Effects Roster Type Species Mycotoxin and Inflammagen formers- version 2.)

The HERTSMI-2 scoring method is a tool to be used in conjunction with the patient's biomarker results, to predict what the total mold burden may be. The scoring of the HERTSMI-2 is a general guideline, and some patients will remain symptomatic even once recommended values are obtained. Building science techniques must be evaluated and optimized as an integral part of the process for the patient to achieve and sustain success.

There are many ways to test for mold and much controversy surrounding mold testing. As of this writing, ONLY the ERMI/HERTSMI-2 test gives a CIRS individual a health/safety exposure result that has been documented. Test results are correlated with specific bio-markers to guide the recovery process. This is why this method is considered among the CIRS community to have the best reliable outcome. Pairing the ERMI and HERTSMI-2 test scoring with a sound building assessment that includes building science methods to mitigate cross contamination, while incorporating a comprehensive CIRS work plan, can move individuals from despair to hope.

Summary for Environmental Testing

There have been, and will continue to be, robust and passionate schools of thought, when discussing environmental testing procedures for the CIRS population. The consensus statement document, 2016 version, (see Resources) states that the qPCR ERMI test is the best and only test that can be used to evaluate the health effects for the CIRS individual. It is the test that is used to discern if the environment is statistically safe to buy, live in, or for re-entry post remediation or cleaning.

The drawback to this test method is that it takes anywhere from two- four weeks to wait for new dust to settle so that the ERMI dust collection can take place, then a few more days for lab processing and results. In the meantime, the environment must stay "isolated" until the results are known. It is for this reason that, while waiting for dust, an alternate option can be to air test using a bio aerosol cassette in each isolated area as a pre qPCR ERMI check. If the air tests fail, then remediation or cleaning can be resumed to correct the problem. This can save time and money in some situations. Once the air tests pass, then wait for dust and perform the ERMI test as per the consensus protocol.

When testing buildings, there are times when it makes sense to use other forms of testing such as tape lifts, microvac testing, inner wall cavity tests, or other testing methods such as ATP testing to determine source locations. These tests are relatively inexpensive and can lead the investigation in the right direction. They do not require invasive action that can potentially cause unnecessary health risk, while adding cost to the client. However, it is critically important to use the endpoint criteria to evaluate the test sample results. (see Appendix)

BUILDING SCIENCE TECHNIQUES

Using appropriate building science techniques is a very important key to CIRS success. Knowing how the various mechanical systems are working within the home can help to identify cross contamination, as well as how mechanical systems are contributing to the health and well-being of the occupants. Carbon monoxide problems are fairly common when gas fired appliances are present. It is imperative that a combustion safety check be done as part of the home assessment. This will ensure that the home's mechanical systems are tested and confirmed to be operating safely.

If there is a furnace and/or air-conditioning system that has a duct system, this system must be evaluated and tested for "duct leakage." This will alert you to potential cross contamination and particulates that can result from a poorly functioning system. If the air conditioning coils are moldy, or the evaporator coil is leaking into the attic space, home performance recommendations can be critical to the ongoing success of the remediation and general health of the home.

Building science can reveal natural occurrences, such as "stack effect", which can contribute to unacceptable indoor air quality. We know that "warm air rises". In winter months, when you are heating your home, the rising warm air, can pull cold air from a number of locations, including a raised crawlspaces lower electrical outlets, and other wall penetrations into the home. The air from a raised crawlspace can harbor a plethora of contaminates. Another cross contaminator can be the use of a "whole house fan". They have the ability to pull large volumes of air through the home by pulling contaminates from unwanted spaces such as crawlspaces, and wall penetrations. The fan housing itself is typically not sealed off from the attic space, which also can allow contaminates into the home from the attic.

The appropriate use of a Heat Recovery Ventilator (HRV) or an Energy Recovery Ventilator (ERV) can have positive health effects. These units add fresh air, while pulling out stale air, in strategic locations. Air sealing techniques are also very beneficial to prevent cross contamination. All of these building science techniques are important factors in creating and maintaining healthy indoor environments, especially for those with CIRS.

Typically, the contractors associated with building science are known as "Home Performance Contractors". **It is the synergistic combination of professional expertise that is able to achieve the comprehensive goal of a Healthy Home**.

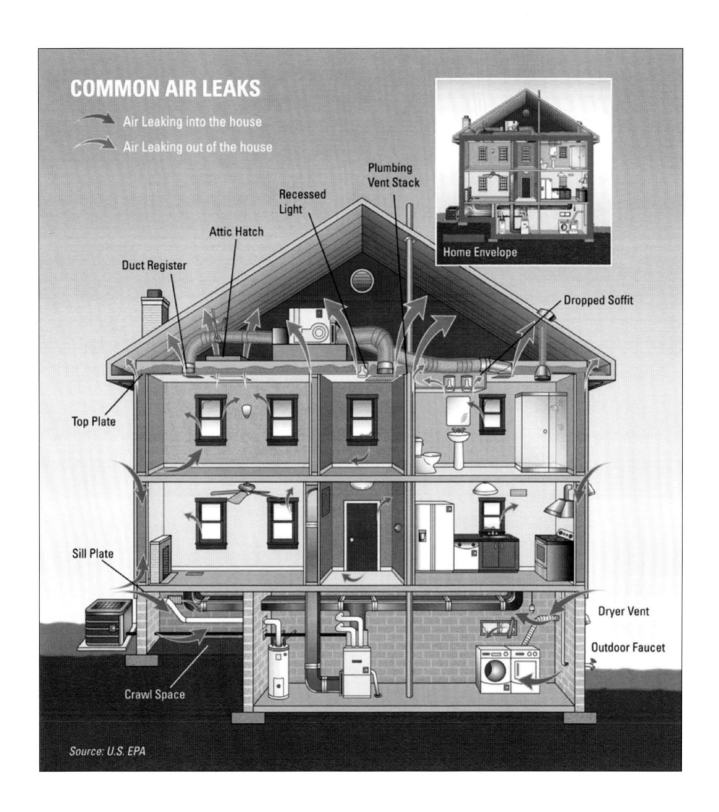

COMMON AIR LEAKS

Air Leaking into the house

Air Leaking out of the house

Home Envelope

Plumbing Vent Stack

Recessed Light

Attic Hatch

Duct Register

Dropped Soffit

Top Plate

Sill Plate

Dryer Vent

Outdoor Faucet

Crawl Space

Source: U.S. EPA

A Husband's "AHA Moment"

My enlightened moment came one evening while I was at an informative meeting in our local city, discussing the topic of *building performance*. I had been feeling overwhelmed after having our home professionally remediated and cleaned, only to find that my wife was still suffering from CIRS. This illness had been so devastating and powerful it had literally drained the life from her and left me feeling absolutely helpless in the process.

Building performance explained the way a home circulates air. Internal and external air pressure can cause particles in the walls and attic to be pulled into the central heating and air conditioner ducts, and then be dispersed throughout a home. That means that molds and other toxins, that you cannot see or smell, can be spread throughout your home or workspace.

Part of the problem with our home was the deterioration of the duct tape used to seal each unit of ductwork. In our home, the leaky ductwork created negative pressure and pulled air into the system from the attic and inner wall cavities. Mold had developed in a wall cavity from a water leak through a crack in the stucco and paper barrier.

Many building performance techniques are utilized to correct these kinds of issues in a home and also create improved energy efficiency. I learned that by making the home more energy efficient, one could actually prevent toxins from being spread through out the home.

This opened my eyes and validated this unseen enemy that was continuing to invade our home and affect Laurie. Before I understood this, I had great difficulty in believing that our home was the cause of her illness, especially after it had been "remediated." Now it started to make sense. With this knowledge, I felt empowered to move forward to have a home where she could become healthy again. From that moment, I was able to more fully support Laurie. I let her know that I was totally on board with whatever needed to be done, because now I understood how important it was to her health and recovery.

CRITICAL ENVIRONMENTAL MANDATES:

Developing a comprehensive action plan involves critical sequential thinking. Most CIRS individuals have "brain fog" due to the inflammation that occurs in the brain. Trying to make sense of this illness is challenging. For most patients and families, the environmental challenges are the hardest to navigate. Having guidance from a CIRS literate environmental professional can save a great deal of time, money and frustration.

Each environmental action plan must be developed from a comprehensive site-specific assessment. Finding resources to perform the various tasks, while following the plan without exception, can be the hardest challenge of all.

The bar is extremely high when making a house safe for a CIRS individual. Emotionally and financially, it needs to be a "one and done" protocol. Most companies that perform standard remediation, cleaning, and construction practices, with standard materials and equipment, simply won't be able to achieve success for the CIRS client. Often, this is because someone on the team didn't think the stringent protocol really needed to be followed **exactly,** and that "corners could be cut."

In our experience, even well experienced and highly competent environmental professionals are not equipped to deal with CIRS unless they have specialized education and training in this illness. What works for 75% of the population, will NOT be adequate for the patient with CIRS.

There must be a system of checks and balances for working through environmental cleaning and remediation. If steps are overlooked or misinterpreted, the patient's health will be jeopardized.

See the Appendix for specific checklists which will familiarize you with various environmental processes and procedures. These include adequate site assessment, remediation, build back, building science techniques known as "home performance contracting" considerations, building cleaning, content cleaning, moving, and proactive maintenance. **You will want a CIRS literate professional to oversee your personalized project, but these checklists will help keep all parties "on the same page."**

These processes are what allow CIRS individuals to transition from just surviving to thriving. This information is an essential component of the roadmap to recovery.

ADDITIONAL TOXINS TO CONSIDER

VOC's (Volatile Organic Compounds) are emitted as gases or vapor from various materials such as paints, varnishes, wax, fuels, organic solvents, disinfectants, plastics, and cosmetic products. There can be as many as ten times the concentration of VOC's inside a home as outside. The VOC gases or vapors will "off-gas" over time but until this happens, the toxicity can contribute to the toxin load in the body and intensify symptoms.

MVOC's (Microbial, Volatile, Organic Compounds) are products of microorganisms such as fungi and bacteria. These microbes "off-gas", releasing certain chemicals into the air. These chemicals can cause severe symptoms in susceptible individuals.

How do VOC's affect CIRS?

Volatile Organic Compounds can complicate the health of the individual as the toxicity from the VOC's can add to the toxic burden. While mold toxins are the primary offender, many individuals with CIRS become increasingly sensitive to VOC's over the course of the disease. Being acutely aware of other forms of toxins that may be affecting your health is important.

A brand new home is usually filled with VOC's and often toxic for a CIRS individual. When buying new household items that are high in VOC's, it is best to allow the product to "off-gas" before bringing the item into the home. There are many products that are certified "low or no VOC" (such as paint) that can be purchased in lieu of the more toxic products. It is important) to read and understand labels, research ingredients, and create your own resources to maintain the lowest toxicity possible.

Live Clean and Avoid Toxins

A healthy resilient body is better able to recover from CIRS. Reducing the TOTAL Toxic Burden in the body will allow detoxification pathways to function more efficiently. In addition to biotoxins, we are exposed to numerous dietary and environmental toxins on a daily basis. While this strategy is not part of the Shoemaker Protocol, it will prepare your body to detoxify and recover with greater ease.

Dietary items to avoid include artificial sweeteners, high fructose corn syrup, MSG, sodas, corn and canola oils, excess sugar, and refined foods full of chemicals!

Rather than compile an endless list of what you should *avoid*, it's far easier to focus on what you should do to lead a CLEAN healthy lifestyle with minimal toxin exposure:

1. As much as possible, buy and eat organic produce and free-range, organic foods to reduce your exposure to pesticides and toxic chemicals. (Check the "dirty dozen" and "clean 15" at EWG.org to see which items are most important to buy organic.)

2. Rather than eating conventional or farm-raised fish, which are often heavily contaminated with PCBs, mercury, and antibiotics, supplement with a high-quality purified fish or krill oil, or eat fish that is wild-caught and lab tested for purity.

3. Eat mostly raw, fresh foods, steering clear of processed, prepackaged foods of all kinds. This way you automatically avoid artificial food additives, including dangerous artificial sweeteners, food coloring and MSG.

4. Store your food and beverages in glass rather than plastic, and avoid using plastic wrap and canned foods (which are often lined with BPA-containing liners). Avoid plastic water bottles.

5. Install a good water filter on your faucets or get a reverse osmosis unit. Drink lots of pure filtered water daily to help flush toxins from your body.

6. Only use natural cleaning products in your home.

7. Switch over to natural brands of toiletries such as shampoo, toothpaste, antiperspirants, sunscreen, and cosmetics. (The Environmental Working

Group has a great database to help you find personal care products that are free of phthalates and other potentially dangerous chemicals.)

8. Avoid using artificial air fresheners, dryer sheets, fabric softeners or other synthetic fragrances.

9. Replace your non-stick cookware with ceramic, glass, or high-grade stainless steel.

10. When redoing your home, look for "green," toxin-free and low VOC alternatives in lieu of regular paint and vinyl floor coverings.

11. Replace your vinyl shower curtain with one made of fabric, or install a glass shower door. Most flexible plastics, like shower curtains, contain dangerous plasticizers like phthalates.

12. Limit your use of drugs (prescription and over-the-counter) as much as possible. Drugs are chemicals too, and they will leave residues and accumulate in your body over time.

13. Avoid spraying pesticides around your home or insect repellants that contain DEET on your body. There are safe, effective and natural alternatives out there.

14. Electrical Magnetic Fields (EMF's) also stress your body and may alter immunity. Do not carry your cell phone in your pocket. Keep it 6 feet from your bed at night when charging. Plug-in alarm clocks should also be at least 6 feet from your bed. Minimize your use of microwave ovens.

15. Get at least 7 hours of sleep each night. Keeping your bedroom cool and totally dark is important.

16. Manage stress in a healthy manner. Deep breathing, prayer, meditation, journaling, art, music can all be helpful.

PREVENTING RE-EXPOSURE

Since 50% of buildings in the US have had water damage, there is a one in two chance that a building entered by a CIRS patient will cause them to become ill. Therefore, it is necessary for the patient to develop time-tested skills in order to avoid being exposed to potentially devastating biotoxins. This allows the patient the opportunity and the choice to be intentional with events that could potentially cause them significant and prolonged illness.

With these critical skills and practices in place, patients are no longer powerless or at the mercy of their circumstances. Instead, patients, family, and friends can successfully navigate around potential exposures with confidence. When you understand that successful avoidance is achievable with a little bit of practice, you find HOPE! You discover the reality that it is possible to gain control over this illness and it no longer has the ability to define or control your life.

Practitioners will tell you to avoid water damaged buildings but how and what does that look like, practically speaking? When you are trying to live out your life with a career, school, family, friends, vacations, medical appointments, and more, you need tools to help you stay safe. It can be extremely difficult when other members of your family, friends, and co-workers are not affected by this illness at all.

Our goal is to provide you with guidelines and tools to use to prevent re-exposure. **Re-exposure awareness** consists of many factors. You may be looking for a new home or rental, deciding if a medical office or grocery store is safe for you to enter, or planning a long awaited vacation with your family. There are spontaneous situations, such as enjoying an afternoon out with friends when they decide to stop at a favorite restaurant to eat. Perhaps you have an important meeting for work, or a parent /teacher conference at a location you are not sure is safe.

You need practical guidelines to prevent re-exposure in a variety of situations. Re-exposure awareness must become "second nature." Being vigilant about your environment can save you countless setbacks. **It is important to remember once you have developed CIRS, with the presence of low MSH, you are at risk of suffering a harmful inflammatory response within as little as ten minutes after being exposed to the interior of a water damaged building.**

It is vital to consider, in advance, the different environments you will encounter when planning a trip, or a drive across town to a new doctor's office or grocery store. Doing so is essential to avoid exposure. It does require additional effort and planning, but yields tremendous benefit when simple steps are taken.

Regularly attended buildings, like a home or workplace, should be tested with an ERMI or HERTSM-2 test as guided by your IEP. It is most likely that mold DNA testing, and or building inspection will not be part of assessment tools for every building a patient plans on entering, due to time frames and expense. Therefore, it is critically important to know what to look for and how to ask for the information you need. This information will allow you to make an educated decision to risk being exposed or not in your day-to-day life.

Staying OUT of exposure will absolutely determine how a patient will progress through CIRS treatment. It also will determine how a patient will benefit from the use of VIP at the top of the protocol. Re-exposure is the biggest hindrance to recovery for the vast majority of patients. The use of VIP can be stopped in its tracks with continued re-exposures. Also, without the use of proper tracking skills, re-exposure is the one thing that can confuse the clinical picture for the patient and practitioner more than any other factor. Re-exposure avoidance must be understood and implemented as a priority.

CRITICAL OBSERVATION SKILLS:

Below are critical observation skills for deciding whether to enter a building based on the acronym MOLDY:

M- Musty smell - If you smell mold or musty smells when you walk in, turn around and leave **IMMEDIATELY**!

O- Old Buildings- There is an extremely high risk of water damage and growth of microbes in older buildings. It is best to avoid them. The best chance of being safe is with buildings between 2 and 12 years old. They represent the least risk if you can verify no water damage has occurred, and "off gassing" of materials used in construction has taken place in newer buildings.

Nearly all older buildings will have had some water intrusion at one point. Older buildings would be considered to be in the 20+ year range. Water damage depends greatly on the quality of materials and type of building practices that were used in the original construction as well as adequate ongoing maintenance of the structure.

L- Look for Leaking – One of the most notorious and easy to spot signs of water intrusion and damage is water stained ceiling tiles. Also, if you look up and there are missing ceiling tiles there is a good chance they have been damaged by water and are being replaced. Look for rippled or buckling floors. Wallpaper may show wrinkling. New paint on part of a wall or ceiling could be hiding a water stain from a leak. Moisture on the inside of a window or door, with or without watermarks, can be a telltale sign.

D- Discoloration- look for discoloration and stains on surfaces, such as wood cabinets, wood ceilings, grout or tile in a bathroom, walls, and ceilings.

Y- Yield to these observations and become diligent in recognizing them! The harsh reality is that, if this kind of tangible evidence is observed in a building, a CIRS patient should not go inside. Entry will more than likely result in re-exposure to mold toxins and predictable setbacks and delays in your treatment progress. The fact is that grocery stores, restaurants, movie theaters, offices, and other commercial buildings must be assumed to be moldy until proven otherwise. You, the patient, will need to be your best advocate in these situations.

If you choose to enter a building you have not been in before, that passes the basic observation skills listed here, it is important to carefully monitor your symptoms for the next few minutes, then over the next 24 to 72 hours. **There are buildings that may not have obvious signs of water damage, but can still expose you to mold toxins and other inflammatory chemicals that produce delayed symptoms. Repeated exposure to "less sick" buildings can still be harmful over time. These buildings pose the most difficult challenge for patients because of the less obvious signs, and the delay in symptoms that occur.**

It is important to track your activity to determine where new or increased symptoms are coming from. If you are not tracking, it is impossible to know if symptoms are due to exposure from a building that has not been entered before, starting/stopping a new medication or supplement, a change in diet, or an exposure to a virus/bacteria. All of these can create an immune response in the CIRS patient. Tracking changes like these is a vital skill that will greatly enhance success with the treatment protocol. (See Tracking form in Appendix.)

NOTE: *As I became aware of these simple observations and put them into practice I was able to effectively eliminate most exposures that I would have suffered from. Early on in my recovery I experienced the thinking and rationalization that, "now that I am better, this won't happen to me." I have watched this thinking happen over and over in many patients when they start to recover and feel better. If I can help patients to understand this important piece of the puzzle, the many pitfalls of re-exposure that can happen with this illness, can be prevented.*

In addition to these basics on what to look for when entering a building, it is also important to know how to ask for information, ahead of time, regarding a building you would like to visit or stay in. One important tip for traveling is: do not stay in any hotel or building that has indoor water features such as fountains, waterfalls, or open terrariums.

TRAVEL with CIRS:

Below are interview guidelines and questions to ask when traveling using the acronym TRAVEL:

T- Talk – Ask to talk with a knowledgeable manager, maintenance person, or someone who knows the history of the building in which you would like to stay or visit at. This could be for a hotel, business, lab, office, or a home of a family or friend. Talking with the individual who has been working or living there the longest period of time will usually be able to give you the information you are looking for.

R- Reaction/Response- When talking to a person with the most knowledge about the building, let them know that **you have a strong and potentially immediate immune reaction/response to any building that has had a water intrusion event or any kind of water damage**. Examples include: problems with plumbing, roof leaks, and fire sprinkler malfunctions, to name a few. Let them know that you realize this can be quite common, and understand that it happens with buildings. **Never ask, "Have you had any problems with mold?" This, unfortunately, puts people on the defensive** because of the liability issues associated with it.

A- Avoid- Let the person you are talking with know you must avoid staying in a building that has had any issues like this to prevent becoming very ill. When approached this way without being critical or demanding, but assertive enough to get the facts you need without judgment, individuals are very helpful in providing you with what you need to know.

V- Validate any Visible signs observed or prior events of water damage that you are being told about, by repeating back to the person you are speaking with what they have described. Ask more about any particular event they have shared. When asked if any water intrusion had occurred, the person responded with: "Not really, we just had a small leak from a plumbing issue with a bathtub that went between the 2nd and 1st floors". Many people assume, unless the water event was a major flood, that these kinds of things don't matter, but they really do for the CIRS patient!

E- Equip yourself with the Evidence you need to make a logical and informed choice about the building you are inquiring about. If you have been given answers by a person who has competent knowledge regarding the building's history that results in no incidences or evidence of water damage, and is a newer structure, your risk of exposure will be significantly less.

L-Let go. If there is no one that is willing or able to talk with you about the history of the building or if any water damage has occurred, it is best to let go and move on to another alternative. If water damage has occurred, there is no real way to verify the kind of efforts that were made to clean, and or remediate to the standards that a CIRS patient requires. With a little more effort, it is possible to find something that is a low risk for exposure instead of settling for a high risk, where an exposure is likely to happen.

It is not easy or convenient to deal with an illness that is caused by the environments you enter. Recognizing and accepting that a "sick building" with water damage will have a negative impact for a CIRS patient plays a huge role in successful management of this illness. Denial of these facts has clearly demonstrated unsuccessful results with recovery.

Practical Example: conversation with a high-end quality hotel

"Hello, I would like to talk with the hotel manager."

"Please hold, I will get the manager for your you."

"Hello, my name is----I am planning on staying in your area, and I need to ask an important question about your hotel before I can make a reservation. I have a medical condition where I can have a severe immune reaction to being inside a building that has had any kind of water intrusion or water damage." "Can you tell me how old the building is?"

"Yes, the building is 4 years old."

"Would you know if this kind of event has occurred recently or in the past in this hotel?"

"I don't think so. I have only been managing here for this last year."

"Is there a maintenance supervisor that knows the history of the building?"

"Yes, please hold while I contact him for you."

"Hello, this is the maintenance supervisor. You had a question regarding water damage?"

"Yes, are you familiar with the history of the hotel?"

"Yes, I have been here since it was built."

"Great. Can you tell me if there has been any history of a water intrusion event at the hotel since it was built?"

"Yes, actually about a year after it was finished there was a malfunction in the fire sprinkler system and it flooded the entire first floor. Everything had to be replaced including the carpet. Everything was repainted as well. It was completely taken care of."

"Thank you, you've been very helpful."

NOTE: This hotel is NOT to be considered safe if you have CIRS!

It is important to realize that even newer buildings can have problems. The only way to know for certain is to ask! If you have been given the information that water damage has taken place, it is NOT the hotel or building for a CIRS patient. In most situations like this, there is no way to be certain how quickly the water event was taken care of or what the hotel did to fix the problem.

Despite the incredible inconvenience that this illness can cause, it is critical to stick to the facts and act on what you know is true. It's normal for the patient and family to want to take shortcuts or skip steps in the environmental diligence required by this illness. Ignoring important clues may be encouraged, by individuals who don't understand the consequences of that decision. This frequently means spending more money, time, and resources and results in delayed recovery, and more heartache for everyone involved.

Preventing Cross Contamination

Cross Contamination is caused by the particulates from the air of a WDB that contain a combination of mold toxins and other inflammatory chemicals. These particulates land on surfaces throughout the affected environment. This includes: furniture, clothing, appliances, window coverings, rugs, flooring, pictures, paper items, etc. In other words, all possessions in a person's home can be affected.

The critical issue is that these particulates that made a person sick inside the water damaged building can then be transferred onto possessions and taken to the new environment without realizing it. This can make a CIRS patient sick in the new building just like it did in the old building.

For this reason, it is mandatory that removal of these particulates take place before moving. **Moving previously contaminated items into the new 'clean" space is one of the most common ways that cross contamination can occur.** This can be one of the most frustrating and costly mistakes made if overlooked.

Cross contamination can also happen when a person, who has previously been in a contaminated environment, then enters a clean environment. Individuals can bring con-taminates with them on their person, clothing, belongings, or other items. Sometimes it may be necessary to create a changing or "decontamination" room to enter from without contaminating the safe environment. (See Appendix)

A patient and their family's daily activities must be evaluated as part of a comprehensive plan to see if these re-exposure risks from cross-contamination are likely. **Cross contamination is a very serious issue and can potentially make the CIRS patient sick without actually living or working in a building that has had water damage.**

Setting up a "decontamination" room, if needed, and paying attention to the details of "Content Cleaning" and "Day to Day Maintenance" will help patients to successfully avoid the hazards of cross contamination. *(See Appendix)*

PACKING TO MOVE OR CLEAN

If you are at this stage of this process, you need to be congratulated for the effort you have made to arrive at this place! It has been a steep climb in a world you previously did not know existed. Many steps have been ones taken when you didn't think you could take one more.

You have navigated through the challenge of understanding the complex medical and environmental information as it applies to CIRS. You have accepted the facts, as they were validated with objective testing, and finally taken action with a treatment protocol for your body and your environment. Both are of equal importance in this illness.

If you have a confirmed diagnosis of CIRS-WDB, and all sources are not removed from your environment, two things will happen:

1. You will not fully recover from CIRS

2. Your practitioner will have much more difficulty in being able to identify the reason your therapy may not be helping you to progress as you should.

At this particular juncture, many patients get cold feet and want to turn back because of the magnitude of what this step entails. Patients will often turn to another professional or a friend who will tell them that this step is "not necessary." This gives them a reason to not have to move forward with this step, and may reinforce a state of denial for the patient and family members. It is very normal to want there to be another way to take care of this problem.

We want to let you know that those who are knowledgeable in this area, as practitioners and environmental professionals, do not take this step lightly when they make their recommendations. **If there were an easier, faster, better, more expedient way possible, to achieve the results needed, it would definitely be used in these circumstances**.

Removal from exposure is the first step in treatment and, for many, the most difficult. We encourage you to think carefully when you arrive at this place. You have one of the most important decisions of your life to make concerning your health if you have been diagnosed with CIRS.

The decision is between recognizing the facts, and the impact that biotoxins have on your health, or denying the facts and continuing to deteriorate from the physical effects.

Many factors in a person's life can affect their perspective when personal items are involved. We recognize this is part of what makes this illness so devastating for patients and their families.

There is no way to minimize the heartache that comes with the realization of potentially having to part with things that have great value and meaning to you. It is never a simple decision to make when it comes to letting go of a home with memories of raising a family, a job that you've worked hard to achieve, a special keepsake from a child, friend, or family member.

It comes down to what really is important. A person's life, their health, and the relationships with those they love and care about is what really matters most. The compromises that are made by going down a "wrong road" repeatedly, and denying what is proven to be true, can be just as responsible for stealing away these important priorities.

The environmental protocol for cleaning, moving, and packing, for CIRS patients, must be followed diligently and in the correct order to be successful. Any attempt to pick and choose which steps to follow, or not to follow, will result in unsuccessful results, potential continued exposure to toxins, and delayed recovery.

By applying the information in this manual, wrong roads can be avoided and the facts will move patients and families to clear action steps that will be successful the first time around. It is important to know that there are options when it comes to your belongings.

The good news is that you don't have to throw away all of your things!

There are specific instructions in the Appendix that will help you decide how to sort through items. They will also help you determine what items can be kept and cleaned and which you will need to let go of.

It's important to know that decisions about what you will keep do not have to be made all at once or right away. Items of great sentimental value you, that you do not know how to clean (or IF they can be cleaned effectively), can be stored in sealed containers until a later time.

Doing this will help you to focus on what needs to be done, in a timely manner, without agonizing over having to part with something that is special to you. This helps move the process along. Many times, there is a way to preserve and keep something that was not originally thought possible.

Practical Example:

Some of my most treasured possessions were pictures and albums of my children growing up. Like many proud parents I kept a few special things they made in school over the years. I knew these things were contaminated and they would not be able to enter our clean environment.

The thought of not having them was devastating to me. I did not have the time or opportunity to spend finding someone to copy them for me. We decided to take that situation off the table completely for a time by storing the pictures and items in a plastic container that we were able to keep at our new home. The outside of this container is clean.

When I am ready, with help, I will take them outside of our clean area and have someone help me take them to be copied or scanned on a computer. I know they are safe where they are and I am not being exposed to them. We took great care to know where they were in the moving process so they did not get misplaced or lost.

I plan to have other things laminated in plastic to preserve them, in a way that will be safe for me to have in our home.

I found, through this process, that the things I thought I could not bear to be without were fewer than I had imagined. We were able to keep most things that had special significance for our family and we learned how to be clutter free.

There is life on the other side of this! All the sacrifice and effort made to eliminate this unseen enemy can bring back what was once taken away by it. Releasing a grasp on things is difficult to do. In these circumstances, it is the only thing to do. Loosening the grasp on those things that are harming you will free you from their devastating effects.

The process of cleaning the inside of a home, or cleaning and sorting personal items, takes time and planning. It can be an arduous task but with a step-by-step action plan, and the right resources, it can be accomplished successfully. *(See Appendix for detailed checklists)*

DAY-TO-DAY MAINTENANCE OF A SAFE LIVING SPACE

Once you have cleaned, remediated, or moved from a water- damaged building, it is extremely important to maintain a clean, toxin free environment. In order to do this, ongoing rigorous cleaning and recognition of potential re-exposures needs to be part of your regular routine.

It is crucial to determine if people living in the "clean" household are coming from a contaminated environment, and take appropriate action. Many patients and family members can easily overlook this step after the huge task of moving or remediating their environment has been completed. This may happen, even when it has been a part of their education, earlier on in the treatment process. Patients and families, at this stage of the process, have usually experienced feeling very overwhelmed on many levels. It is normal to feel the desire for "this to end" at some point.

We want to assure patients that successful day-to-day maintenance is possible with the awareness and implementation of certain safeguards. Without these precautions, it is probable that cross contamination will occur to the point where levels of toxins inhibit their recovery. It is important to remember, **"particulates from the air of any water damaged building that you transfer onto yourself or your possessions will make you sick in the new building just like they did in the old building."**

If it has been determined that a husband, wife, child, or anyone living in the "clean house" is working, attending, or frequenting a building on a regular basis that is known or suspected to be contaminated, it is important to consider having a changing room or decontamination area. This is a designated space, **outside of the "safe" environment,** that will allow people to enter the home without contaminating the clean environment.

A decontamination area can vary in size, and complexity depending on the amount and type of incoming source(s). Weather is also an important factor. Creating a decontamination area in Montana, where the air is dry with low humidity with extreme temperatures can be 20 below zero, will have different considerations than Florida, where high humidity and a mild climate will require a different decontamination area plan. (See decontamination considerations in the Appendix)

Practical Example:

My family and I felt great relief after moving to a newly constructed home designed and built to avoid water damage. After going through the painstaking process of content cleaning and moving into our new home, we thought we were free of these invisible culprits called biotoxins that had taken over our lives. We were also mentally, emotionally, and physically exhausted from the process. What we failed to acknowledge, at this point, is the amount of toxins that could potentially be coming from my husband's workplace during this transition period.

His workplace had not been tested because we felt that our home, having been water damaged, was "the source" of toxins causing the problem. What we were not aware of was that his office, once tested, was also a source of three problematic molds and their associated toxins. This means that we had gotten rid of one source of the problem, but in reality, there was more than one continuous source of toxins. This source would be considered to be from "cross-contamination."

How did we know? We ERMI tested once we had done a post construction cleaning and moved all of the cleaned items into the home. We verified that our efforts with diligent moving precautions had been successful. We had a clean baseline from that point.

After 3 months in the home we tested again with a HERTSMI-2 and were shocked to find the three mold species inside our new home. These were the exact species that were confirmed in my husband's office. It was hard to believe that the test numbers we saw in our brand new home, with no water damage and a previous negative DNA test, were from cross contamination alone!

It is important to acknowledge that Cross Contamination alone, regardless of the source, may cause a CIRS patient to remain ill, and prevent them from progressing through the treatment steps.

With that information, we had to find a way to for my husband return from his work (a now known contaminated source) and enter our clean home without continuing to cross contaminate it and re-expose me to mold toxins and contaminates.

A "Decontamination Area" or "Changing Space" was established in a location outside our home where he could remove his outer clothing and shoes and put them into a container. A clean change of clothes was available to put on and enter the home with. All items from that contaminated environment were not allowed into our clean space. Used clothes are deposited directly into a washing machine through a plastic bag that has been sealed and opened only once inside the washing machine. This laundry room has a door that closes off to the rest of the house. We put HEPA filtration inside this room and have an exhaust fan that pulls air up and out of the room, to prevent any contaminates from re-circulating.

After cleaning and re-testing, the HERTSMI-2 was back to the original clean baseline result. This is not an uncommon situation and has been reported with other patients where **cross-contamination was coming from the children's school environment after the home was shown to be safe** with appropriate environmental testing. With one particular case, the patient found that VIP was no longer effective for her. The patient's lab work showed elevation of inflammatory markers and worsening in VCS testing, even though this patient was not going anywhere outside her confirmed clean environment.

Similarly, a decontamination area was set up for the children and their school items. The patient was able to resume taking the VIP with benefit. Her inflammatory markers and VCS testing improved once more, and she has continued to make progress on her road to recovery.

It is crucial to not only know "who" is coming in the home and where they have been, but also "what" is coming in to the home and "where" it came from.

It is important to acknowledge that there is a potential for cross-contamination by bringing items into your home from outside various sources other than a regular workplace or school environment. For this reason, it is important to consider these situations below, once you have established a safe environment.

People who will be entering your home need to be prepared in advance with information they need to help keep a CIRS patient safe. This helps friends and family know what to expect and reduces anxiety on everyone's part about what needs to take place. They can arrive prepared and many awkward moments can be avoided. Once these steps are acknowledged and understood to be crucial, implementation can become part of your routine activities.

If one has a "clean" or "non-contaminated" item and takes it to a "dirty" or "contaminated" area, the item becomes "dirty." If one has a "dirty" item and takes it into a "clean" area, that clean area becomes "dirty" or "contaminated." It is important to assess your situations and determine if the item is clean or dirty, and if the environment you are taking things to or from is clean or dirty. If you take a few moments to think about what you are doing, it is clear what to do next and what not to do. If this concept is learned and practiced, it can save an enormous amount of time, cleaning, and frustration! Always remember the home you have painstakingly cleaned and or re mediated and cleared for toxins is considered "clean." The challenge is keeping it that way.

Although this is a simple concept it is not always easy to implement with all that goes on during moving, cleaning, and the amount of people that may be involved helping with this process. Organizing and explaining this to those that are helping will greatly reduce the amount of errors with accidental contamination of clean items, and help to avoid having to re-clean an area contaminated by a dirty item in this process.

Practical Example:

#1. When we were in temporary housing that was verified clean, my husband brought a desk into that clean space. That desk, although initially not contaminated, was being stored with other items brought over from our contaminated home. The "dirty" items from our home made the storage room "contaminated" along with everything in it! The desk was promptly removed and cleaned properly!

#2. In our new home the garage is attached to the house. This is a very common floor plan. There is a back door in the house that enters into the garage and then a door in the garage that exits outside. It is important to understand that the clean area of your home extends to the garage in this kind of floor plan. Placing contaminated items in the garage can allow contaminates to enter the home. Since our garage is considered "clean", "dirty" items cannot enter into it. The likelihood of cross contaminating the inside of our home becomes very probable if we do not pay VERY close attention to this detail.

Examples of Potential Sources of Contaminates Entering Your Home and Instructions for Managing Them:

1. Packages being delivered by mail

Remove new sealed items from their shipping boxes before bringing into the home.

2. Groceries and store bought items

It is possible that a family member may bring home items from a store that is contaminated. If this should occur, it is important to wash newly purchased clothing or clean items before exposing them to your safe environment.

Grocery items should be removed from bags and any packaging that might be contaminated before bringing them into the clean environment.

3. Items brought to a home by family members and friends

If a family member or friend is coming to stay with you and is known to live in a contaminated building, bringing porous items such as a fabric suitcase or backpack could cause cross-contamination to occur. Leather (not suede) or vinyl smooth surfaces can be wiped down prior to entering. Backpacks can be washed in a washing machine before coming into the "clean" space. **If it is not known if the building, where guests are coming from, is contaminated, these precautions must be an active part of preventing re-exposure for the CIRS patient.** Clothing brought or worn by family, friends, or guests should be freshly laundered and put on just prior to leaving their own environment and entering your clean environment.

4. Outer clothing such as jackets, shoes, purses, backpacks

The bottoms of shoes are considered to be some of the most contaminated items a person owns. For this reason, **shoes must be taken off before entering and kept out of the safe environment. This can be outside or in a designated changing space for contaminated items. This includes shoes of the occupants of the home and anyone who enters the home.**

Outer jackets or coats that are not washed or dry cleaned, along with fabric bags, purses, and backpacks, need to be placed in a designated space outside of the safe home before entering. Note: Is the dry cleaning building safe?

5. **Traveling in a car** that has been used by a person who routinely is in a contaminated environment (or unknown to be in a clean environment) can be a source of re-exposure.

Taking your own vehicle whenever possible is the best option. If you are a CIRS patient that has cleaned, remediated, and or moved, please understand that cleaning and maintaining your car is an important step to prevent potential re-exposure.

Practical Example:

My husband works in a known contaminated building and routinely drives his truck to and from the office. After moving to our safe home and knowing his vehicle was new, attention was not given to the possibility of me being exposed in this way. Over time, I was able to determine, with tracking my symptoms, which ones would appear after being inside his vehicle. At this time, I was not nearly as reactive to mold toxins after using VIP. However, **repeated exposure to a confirmed source of toxins and contaminates over time can still have adverse effects on a CIRS patient's health.**

For me to be able to use or ride in this particular vehicle, without eventually being negatively affected, it must be HEPA vacuumed and wiped down thoroughly beforehand. When these precautions are performed adequately, along with routinely tracking symptoms, re-exposures from these situations can be avoided.

If there has been water damage inside a vehicle that has not been remediated properly, it can be a source of exposure. Addressing it as a known source of toxins is necessary, if confirmed. Certain things can be cleaned while in some situations the car may need to be replaced. It is important to have help in identifying the facts about what truly exists in your particular situation.

The heating, cooling and ventilation systems in a car can become compromised, just as they can in a building, due to water damage. For trucks/SUV's especially, where they have been, and what they have hauled can make them contaminated. For example, just as mold and other contaminates can be found in the evaporator coil of an air conditioner in the home, so can they be found in the evaporator core and duct system in a car or truck.

What routine activities and checks need to be performed in your home on a regular basis to prevent a potential water damage situation from occurring?

Certain items in a home need to be consistently and routinely checked, as you use them, for malfunctions, leaks, or other problems. It is helpful to put these activities on a checklist and give specific time frames when they need to be done. Check them off when completed. This allows the best opportunity to prevent a problem from escalating and causing significant damage. (See Appendix for Household Proactive Maintenance Checklist)

During the winter or rainy seasons, this activity should be stepped up because of the higher probability of water damage during this time. **Regular maintenance, fixing problems as soon as they appear, and being aware of possible breaches in the building envelope, can go a long way in preventing a major problem down the road.**

It is important to develop the habit of looking at these items as a part of your daily routine. Other things that you don't have contact with every day can be put on a schedule for regular checks. This may include the furnace, HVAC system, ducting systems, and filter changes.

1. Plumbing fixtures: toilets, under all sinks, showers, clothes washer, dish washer, refrigerators and automatic ice makers, and hot water heaters. Any indication of water leaking from these areas needs to be addressed immediately. Appliance alarms can be purchased for about $18.00 each. These can be put under sinks, dishwashers, and behind refrigerators with icemakers. They will sound an alarm when they sense moisture.

2. Any fans that are installed to eliminate moisture, such as in bathrooms and laundry rooms, need to be functioning correctly. They should have a moisture sensor to turn on and off when high humidity or moisture is detected. (See Rebuilding for CIRS in the Appendix)

3. Periodic checks need to be scheduled for furnace, air conditioning units, attic and crawlspace areas.

4. HVAC filters need to be changed on a regular basis.

5. All windows and doors need to be routinely inspected for problems with possible leaks or problems with sealing.

6. Flooring needs to be routinely inspected for moisture problems.

7. Periodic duct work inspection and cleaning needs to be scheduled.

8. Check all roof penetrations and general condition of roofing components, such as chimney flashing, roof to wall metal, plumbing vents, flashing, and skylights. Make sure all penetrations are well sealed. Inspect fascia and roof overhang materials to ensure the materials are not degrading, cracked, or peeling. A good coat of paint is your first line of protection on the roof overhangs and eaves.

Practice proactive maintenance in lieu of reactive maintenance.

Ongoing rigorous cleaning efforts must include:

- Weekly HEPA vacuuming of floors and sofas
- Weekly dusting of surfaces with microfiber cloths
- Weekly wet mop floors
- It is important to AVOID clutter as much as possible. Clutter collects dust particles. This is where particulates from fragments of mold, microbes, and chemicals often end up.

Once or Twice yearly:

Whole house cleaning or fogging depending on amount of activity going on in the home. *(See Appendix for details)*

Decontamination Room

CIRS individuals and families must implement a "decontamination plan" to reduce any cross contamination that will pose a health risk. There are several considerations, most of which are contained within this manual. However, there may be instances where the incoming contamination is such that it is imperative to create an ancillary method of reducing cross contamination at the point of entry to a home. Here is one practical real life example that was created due to the harsh weather conditions. In a more temperate climate, where cross contamination is likely, outer clothing and shoes may be removed and kept in bins outdoors, to be safely stored until needed.

Example: A family lives on a ranch in Wyoming. The child goes to a school, father works on the ranch, mother is CIRS activated and not improving as she should be. Wyoming winter is coming. The temperature drops and wind chill is such that removing outer clothing, before coming into the house, is not an option.

The answer was to build an ancillary room, within the garage space, that was designed to work as a decontamination area. This included an air lock, using positive and negative air flows, as appropriate, to create a chamber where contaminates could be stopped within the first chamber. Outer clothing, shoes, back-packs, etc. were removed in this area. The individual then moved to another chamber to put on "house clothes" and come into the home. Creating this type of "decontamination system" for CIRS individuals and families has made a significant difference between *Surviving and Thriving*.

TIPS TO THRIVE WITH CIRS

Over years of educating and advocating for clients with CIRS, certain consistencies have become apparent. **There are specific attitudes and behaviors, which predict which patients will move steadily forward on the road to recovery and which will likely get "detoured" repeatedly.**

Take a good hard look at these predictors. Can you benefit from adjustments in your own treatment, diligence, or attitude? Committing to what we **know works**, will make the difference between success and failure. It's your time to THRIVE!

Those who "get stuck" or find recurring "detours":

Do not accept the facts of their illness. Denial is powerful. Some will search for other diagnoses, even when their genetic test, biomarkers, clinical symptoms & environmental testing conclusively show CIRS.

Are non-compliant with CIRS treatment protocol. CIRS is not a convenient diagnosis, but following the protocol **precisely** is the key to success. The protocol won't work if you don't work the protocol!

Ignore the impact of multiple indoor environments. Refusal to get OUT of exposure & refusal to practice awareness techniques to avoid re-exposures is self-defeating. Ignoring the importance of remediation and cleaning practices, in order to make environment safe, will prevent recovery.

Are unwilling to track changes in symptoms, environments entered, activity level, starting or stopping any medications or supplements, diet, treatments, etc. Without accurate tracking, exposure prevention is much more difficult.

Add multiple interventions (supplements, dietary changes, medications, treatments) all at once, or in a random fashion, without keeping track of anything. When making multiple changes at once, we don't know what is helping or hindering.

Are not consistent or disciplined in their treatment regimen. Each step of the protocol has a scientific reason. To "pick and choose," or to do the steps out of sequence, will undermine their effectiveness.

Avoid asking for support or accepting support when it is offered.

Those who predictably move forward to THRIVE:

Understand their illness and how it affects their body.

Accept the facts of their case, demonstrated by appropriate objective testing.

Comply with their treatment protocol. Be consistent and disciplined with your treatment plan and stick with it for a definite period of time before changing or adding anything to the mix.

Understand that environmental exposure MUST be avoided. Make necessary environmental changes, with knowledgeable guidance.

Track changes routinely to improve their health including: symptoms, environments entered, activity level, starting or stopping any medications or supplements, diet, treatments, etc.

Implement one thing at a time and only one new thing at a time.

Get support when needed.

RESOURCES

CERTIFIED CIRS PRACTITIONERS: (Shoemaker Protocol)
www.SurvivingMold.com

READING: (e-books available on www.SurvivingMold.com)
Mold Warriors (2005) by Dr. Ritchie Shoemaker

Surviving Mold (2010) by Dr. Ritchie Shoemaker

"Owls Under the Beaver Moon" (2014) Essay
Dr. Ritchie Shoemaker www.SurvivingMold.com

State of the Art Questions to 500 Mold Questions by
Dr. Ritchie Shoemaker www.SurvivingMold.com

Desperation Medicine (2001) by Dr. Ritchie Shoemaker

The Brain on Fire (2014) Paper by Dr. Mary Ackerley
www.survivingmold.com

CIRS OFFICIAL WEBSITE:(Dr. Ritchie Shoemaker - Surviving Mold)
www.SurvivingMold.com

DVDs & VIDEOs:
www.SurvivingMold.com "store"

www.youtube.com (search Surviving Mold or Dr. Ritchie Shoemaker)

https://vimeopro.com/cornerstonemediapro/surviving-mold

Patient Interviews: "CIRS Answers for Hope and Healing"
1. **http://vimeo.com/75808458** password: biotoxin
2. **http://vimeo.com/80853158** password: biotoxin

ONLINE COURSE:
Mold Illness Made Simple - Dr. Sandeep Gupta (Australia)
www.moldillnessmadesimple.com

SUPPORT GROUP: (Telephone)
Patti Schmidt: **pattischmidtcoaching.com** pattisch@me.com

ENVIRONMENTAL TESTING KITS:
www.Mycometrics.com (ERMI & HERTSMI-2)
www.Envirobiomics.com (ERMI & HERTSMI-2)

ENVIRONMENTAL PROFESSIONALS:(CIRS Literate)
See **www.survivingmold.com**
Indoor Environmental Professionals Consensus Statement
(Schwartz, L. et al) in References

ENVIRONMENTAL SUPPLIES: (cleaning, filters, masks, etc.)
Cleaning products:
Benefect- **www.benefect.com**
Concrobium Mold control- **www.concrobium.com**
On Guard cleaner- **http://www.tryessentialoil.com/wp-content/uploads/downloads/2012/09/OnGuardCleanerConcentrate.pdf**
Borax- Effective cleaner such as 20 mule team brand. Combine 1 cup of borax to 1 gallon of water. (1:16 ratio) Found in laundry aisle of grocery.

Quaternary cleaners- 409 household cleaner & Fantastic household cleaner.

Wipes- Swiffer cloths, bucket 'o towels, anti-static Swiffer cloths.

NOTE: *Studies have shown that using microfiber cloths combined with a quaternary compound for mold removal is much less effective and is not recommended. If microfiber cloths are to be used, then it is best to use a peroxide based cleaner in lieu of a quaternary cleaner.*

Cold Fogging products:

Aerosolver - **www.aerosolver.com**

Concrobium "mold control." **www.concrobium.com**

Mold remediation products:

CMSR (Concrobium Mold Stain Remover) Use PPE (Personal Protective Equipment) **www.concrobium.com**

Shockwave by Fiberlock/use PPE

Benefect- **www.benefect.com**

Esporta machine: http://www.esporta.us/home.html

Household HEPA vacuum: Meets minimum HEPA vacuum requirements. Miele S6290 Jasper.

HEPA Back Pack Vacuum: http://www.amazon.com/Atrix-VACBP1-Hepa-Backpack

Tacky Mats: https://www.uline.com/BL_1762/Clean-Mats

AIR PURIFIER: These units are to be used to help facilitate daily maintenance in a clean environment, NOT as a replacement for remediation or to reduce toxins if there is a mold presence. There is much ongoing research in the technology and clinical effects of air purification in CIRS.

A true **HEPA Air Purifier** can be helpful. We do not recommend air purifiers that use Ozone and/or UV lights. Nothing we have found replaces the processes within this manual for a WDB.

Airfree purifiers **www.http://www.airfree.com/en-US/home-page.aspx** It will incinerate the mold and spores with an internal temperature of 400 degrees. This has a positive effect with mold bacteria, viruses, and overall particulate matter and some VOC success with low level VOC's.

FURNACE FILTERS: MERV 13 pleated type filter.

BUILDING PERFORMANCE Institute: www.bpi.org

Face mask- P- 100

http://respro.com/store/product/respro-allergy-mask

MARCoNS TESTING:

Microbiology DX: **www.microbiologydx.com** 781-276-4956

COMPOUNDING PHARMACIES: (CIRS Literate)

Hopkinton: **www.rxandhealth.com** (508) 435-4441

Woodland Hills: **www.woodlandhillspharmacy.com** (818) 876-3060

REFERENCES

Al-Mutairi D, Kilty SJ. Bacterial biofilms and the pathophysiology of chronic rhinosinusitis. *Current Opinion in Clinical Allergy and Immunology*. 2011 Feb;11(1):18-23.

Berndtson K, McMahon S, Ackerley M, Rapaport S, Gupta S & Shoemaker RC (2015). Medically sound investigation and remediation of water-damaged buildings in cases of CIRS-WDB: Consensus Statement Part 1. **www.survivingmold.com**

B.P.I. (Building Performance Institute), Inc. Building Analyst Professional Training Handbook. (2005)

Campbell A, Thrasher J, Gray M & Vojdani A. Mold and mycotoxins: effects on the neurological and immune systems in humans. Advances in Applied Microbiology. 2004;55: 375-406.

Candelario-Jalil E, Thompson J, Taheri S, Grossetete M, et al. Matrix metalloproteinases are associated with increased blood-brain barrier opening in vascular cognitive impairment. *Stroke*. 2011 Mar 31.

Catania A, Caterina L, Sordi A, Carlin A, Leonardi P, Gatt S. The melanocortin system in control of inflammation. *The Scientific World Journal* 2010;10:1840-1853.

Delgado M, Gonzalez-Rey E, Ganea D. Vasoactive intestinal peptide. *Annals of the New York Academy of Sciences*. 2006 Aug 2;1070:233-238.

Gray, M. Molds and mycotoxins: beyond allergies and asthma. Alternative Therapies in Health and Medicine. 2007;13: 5146-5152.

Karunasena E, Larrañaga MD, Simoni JS, Douglas DR, Straus DC. Building-Associated Neurological Damage Modeled in Human Cells: A Mechanism of Neurotoxic Effects by Exposure to Mycotoxins in the Indoor Environment. Mycopathologia. 2010 Jun 13.

Kriegel MA, Ming LO, Sanjabi S, Wan YY, Flavell RA. Transforming growth factor-beta: recent advances on its role in immune tolerance. *Current Rheumatology Reports*. 2006;8:138-144.

Krigger, J. (2013) Residential Energy: Cost Savings and Comfort for Existing Buildings (6th Ed)

Lipton JM, Catania, A. Mechanisms of anti-inflammatory action of the neuroimmunomodulatory peptide alpha-MSH. PMID: 12470216

Luger TA, Scholzen TE, Brzoska T, Bohm, M. New insights into the functions of alpha- MSH and related peptides in the immune system. PMID: 12851308

McMahon, SW, Shoemaker RC, & Ryan JC. (2016) Reduction in forebrain parenchymal and cortical grey matter swelling across treatment groups in patients with inflammatory illness acquired following exposure to water-damaged buildings. Journal of neuroscience and clinical research, 2016,1(1).

Olfert IM, Howlett RA, Tang K, Dalton ND, et al. Muscle-specific VEGF deficiency greatly reduces exercise endurance in mice. *Journal of Physiology*. 2009 Apr 15;587:1755- 1767.

Pestka J, Zhou HR. Toll-like receptor priming sensitizes macrophages to proinflammatory cytokine gene induction by deoxynivalenol and other toxicants. *Toxicological Science*. 2006 Aug;92(2):445-455.

Pinto, Michael. (2004). Mold clean-up projects: Post remediation criteria are critical to success. Professional Safety. Nov. 2004.

Pinto, Michael. (2008). 2nd edition. Fungal Contamination, A Comprehensive Guide for Remediation.

Schwartz L, Weatherman G, Schrantz M, Spakes W, Charlton J, Berndston K & Shoemaker RC (2016). Indoor environmental professionals panel of surviving mold – Consensus Statement. **www.survivingmold.com**

Shoemaker RC, Hudnell HK. Possible estuary associated syndrome: symptoms, vision and treatment. Environmental Health Perspectives. 2001 May; 109 (5): 539-545.

Shoemaker RC. Differential association of HLADR genotypes with chronic neurotoxin mediated illness: possible genetic basis for susceptibility. American Journal of Tropical Medicine. 2002;67 (2): 160.

Shoemaker R, Hudnell D. A time-series study of sick building syndrome: chronic, biotoxin-associated illness from exposure to water-damaged buildings. Neurotoxicology and Teratology 2004; 1-18.

Shoemaker RC, Schaller J, Schmidt P. (2005) Mold Warriors: Fighting America's Hidden Threat. Gateway Press: Baltimore.

Shoemaker RC, Rash J & Simon E. Sick building syndrome in water-damaged buildings: generalization of the chronic biotoxin associated illness paradigm to indoor toxigenic fungi. Bioaerosols, fungi, bacteria, mycotoxins and human health. Eckardt Johanning MD editor 2006.

Shoemaker R, House D. Sick building syndrome (SBS) and exposure to water- damaged buildings: Time series study, clinical trial and mechanisms. Neurotoxicology and Teratology 2006; 573-588.

Shoemaker R, Giclas P, Crowder C & House D. Complement split products C3a and C4a are early markers of acute Lyme disease in tick bite patients in the United States. International Archives of Allergy Immunol 2008; 146: 255-261.

Shoemaker R. Exposure to water damaged buildings causes a readily identifiable chronic inflammatory response syndrome successfully treated by a sequential intervention protocol. Biology of Fungi, International Mycology Congress 2009 (conference peer review)

Shoemaker RC. (2010) Surviving Mold: Life in the Era of Dangerous Buildings. Otter Bay Books: Baltimore.

Shoemaker RC, Mark L, McMahon S, et al. Policyholders of America research committee report on diagnosis and treatment of chronic inflammatory response syndrome caused by exposure to the internal environment of water-damaged buildings. 2010 July: 1-161.

Shoemaker RC, House DE & Ryan JC. (2010) Defining the neurotoxin derived illness chronic ciguatera using markers of chronic systemic inflammatory disturbances: a case study. Neurotoxicology and teratology, 32(6), 396-401.

Shoemaker RC. ACOEM position statements on mold: ploys and lies. Published on line 2011.

Shoemaker R, House D, Ryan J. Vasoactive intestinal polypeptide (VIP) corrects chronic inflammatory response syndrome (CIRS) acquired following exposure to water- damaged buildings. Health 2013; 3: 396-401.

Shoemaker RC, House DE & Ryan JC (2014). Structural brain abnormalities in patients with inflammatory illness following exposure to water-damaged buildings: a volumetric MRI study using NeuroQuant. Neurotoxicology and teratology (45) 18-26.

Shoemaker RC, Katz D, Ackerley M, Rapaport S, McMahon S, Berndtson K, Ryan JC (2017). Intranasal VIP safely restores volume to multiple grey matter nuclei in patients with CIRS. Internal Medicine Review (April 2017)

Vesper S, McKinstry C, Haugland R, Wymer L, et al. Development of an environmental relative moldiness index for U.S. homes. Journal of Environmental Medicine. 2007 Aug;49(8): 829-833.

APPENDIX

DISCLAIMER

ENVIRONMENTAL

The standard for mold remediation is extremely high for clients with CIRS. Many experienced and otherwise qualified mold remediators are not familiar with the specific stringent requirements that apply to CIRS. For this reason, we have included very detailed checklists. These are to be used **with** your Indoor Environmental Professional (IEP) in designing and implementing a comprehensive work plan that is successful.

These checklists are NOT to be used to carry out a "do it your-self" project. The expertise required to accomplish a successful remediation, without catastrophic cross-contamination, is substantial.

A tiny breach in a single step of the process can result in an epic FAIL. We have seen tens of thousands of dollars wasted by well-meaning clients who attempted to 'fix it myself." Professional guidance by a CIRS literate environmental expert is essential to provide for your specific needs.

BUILDING CLEANING

GENERAL GUIDELINES CHECKLIST

This can be used to review with IEP, Cleaning/Remediation company.

Client name:

_____

Site address:

_____

Date Remediation completed:

_____

Date of Post- Remediation clearance:

_____

Build back complete: yes/no

_____

Building science/home performance techniques completed yes/no

_____

_____

_____

Has the HVAC or furnace system been tested for mold? Y N

Has the ducting and evaporator coil (if applicable) been cleaned? Y N

Any rooms in isolation? Y N

_____

Why?

_____

_____

_____

_____

Other remarks:

_____

_____

_____

Remove all contents from the home for the best results. (I e. food, dishes, clothes, furnishings, window coverings... stuff) out of the home.

Note: For long term, optimum results for the CIRS individual it is best to remove and replace carpeting with a solid surface flooring. Carpet can become or remain a "reservoir" of contaminates. Rugs, on the other hand, can be used to help leave contaminates at the entry ways. A small rug is easier to remove and launder on a frequent basis than trying to keep wall to wall carpet clean.

☐ Carpet/Rugs

☐ Contents

☐ Paper

☐ Kitchen dishes

☐ Food

☐ All cabinets cleaned out

_____

☐ Beds

_____

☐ Furniture

_____

☐ Items that stay to be covered and cleaned in room

_____

☐ Drapes, windows, coverings, blinds

_____

☐ Pictures, art

_____

Correction/comments:

_____

_____

_____

_____

Cleaning plan sequence for the interior of the home.

Step one:

Identify any designated "clean" rooms within the building. (Rooms that have been tested/proven as safe and will be used to store cleaned items).

Room 1: _____ barriers intact? Y N

Date cleared:

_____

Room 2: _____ barriers intact? Y N

Date cleared:

_____

Room 3: _____ barriers intact?   Y   N

Date cleared:

_____

Step two: Room set up

☐ Open a window. (weather permitting, attach tackified filter in window vent.)

☐ Isolate doorways/critical barriers each room, hallway, etc.

☐ Tacky mats before entry.

☐ Set negative pressure in each room to be cleaned.

☐ Turn off HVAC/ protect sensors and equipment.

☐ Seal off with two layers all furnace or HVAC supply and return grilles.

☐ Air scrubbers in each room as cleaned.

☐ Clean and cover/seal any items that must be left in room.

☐ Clean staged equipment left outside.

☐ Bring in cleaned equipment, supplies.

Step three: Room cleaning process

☐ HEPA vacuum the entire room (start at the furthest away from the door on the ceiling, clean towards the door and position the intake of the air scrubber (with diffuser tail) intake facing toward the cleaning process), HEPA vacuum the walls in same sequence, then floors in same sequence (farthest from the doorway working to the doorway.)

☐ Wet wipe the entire room using "exposure tested" patient tolerable product (see appendix product resource list) start with ceiling first far corner to room exit, follow same method for walls, far corner to exit, then wipe floors, far corner to exit. Let dry.

☐ Air scrub (with diffuser tail) keeping the intake facing toward the cleaning process while wet wiping depending on size of air scrubber and room for air changes. (See appendix resource list for equipment and detailed instructions).

Optional method: If surfaces are rough or not accessible, start air wash (using clean leaf blower powered by electric or battery). Perform similar sequence, high areas to low areas into HEPA air scrubber intake. If leaf blower is used, then HEPA vacuum the entire room again.

☐ Small particle cleaning must be performed by applying the cold fogging technique described in the consensus document using "exposure tested" patient tolerable product (see appendix product environmental resource list).

☐ If built in cabinets, such as kitchen cabinets, are in the room to be cleaned, then use the "HEPA vacuum, wet wipe, allow to dry" method of cleaning for the cabinet interior.

☐ Upon completion of the room cleaning, it is extremely important to perform a visual and "white glove" test, which can be a "swiffer cloth" along surfaces within the room. If there is visual dust on the "swiffer cloth", then re clean until no visual dust is present on a "swiffer cloth" or "white glove".

☐ Close open windows, remove equipment from room, and seal doorway to isolate from other rooms to await testing for contaminates.

Step four: Post cleaning visual walk through:

☐ PASS ☐ FAIL

Remarks:

_____

_____

If the visual walk through is a **pass**, then you can either wait the typical 2-3 weeks for dust to gather for collecting using a qPCR ERMI test while rooms are kept sealed in isolation, or another option is to perform a bio aerosol test for "initial" quick test results. The turnaround time for the air test can be a couple of days to a week depending on the lab. Getting quick initial test results will allow you to re clean immediately in lieu of waiting three weeks for dust to collect in a room only to find out that it was a fail. The initial bio aerosol test does NOT replace the ERMI, it only serves to gain time and money in some situations where it makes sense to do so.

Initial quick pre-testing method:

Air testing: Pass or Fail (see endpoint criteria in the appendix resource list)

Maintain room seal during and after testing.

If initial quick bio aerosol pre-test fails: Check procedures, verify that all sources have been removed or remediated. Go back to step two and re clean until you can pass the initial testing.

If initial quick pre-test passes: Keep room isolated until qPCR ERMI testing (dust sampling) can be completed, test results known. **(Remember to wait about 2-3 weeks for enough dust to accumulate for the ERMI sampling).**

Step five: Upon receiving qPCR ERMI dust test results, send the results to your practitioner to score using the HERTSMI-2 scoring method. The HERTSMI-2 scoring along with the practitioner's input will give you a health risk determination and recommendation for a pass to move in after content cleaning, or if the result is a fail, reassess the situation.

CARPET REMOVAL INSTRUCTIONS

Work from the farthest room in the back toward the front of the home (typically). The idea is to work your way out of the home without having to go back into a cleaned room.

In each room: Work in a corner farthest away from the door, and from the top down.

Remove everything from the room(s) including drapes, blinds, blind hardware, clothes, furniture, everything.

If supply registers are in the floor, remove the grilles and use a HEPA vacuum to vacuum out the duct. Seal off all supply or return registers in the room taping off the opening to prevent contamination during the process.

Stage your removal supplies, which would include a spritz spray bottle or new garden sprayer, carpet knife, hammer and crow bar to remove the tack strip, trash bags, HEPA vacuum, HEPA Negative Air Machine(NAM) etc.

Enter room, shut door and seal with 6mil plastic sheeting, taped /stapled to the outside edge of the door casing. There should be a zipper in the middle of the doorway to create a barrier with appropriate access from the other rooms during the process.

Set up HEPA negative air machine (NAM) to use as an air scrubber during this process and turn on. The NAM should be pointed towards the work to remove any aerosolized particles, spores etc.

HEPA vacuum entire room.

Cut carpet in 3 foot to 4 foot strips.

Spray carpet or spritz with water using a spray bottle or clean garden type sprayer. Do not drench. The purpose is to help keep the dust down while removing the carpet.

Roll up the carpet strips and dispose into a doubled trash bag. Seal the top of the bag via "Goose neck", twisted and taped to eliminate contamination during removal transport.

Take bags out through a window, if possible, rather than through the house. HEPA vacuum and wet wipe the outside of the trash bag using a pretested product such as "Benefect," Mold Control, or similar product (see resource list) if taking through the house before disposal.

Repeat the same process with the carpet pad.

Remove the tack strip and place in bags with the nails toward the inside so as not to tear the bag. Remove from the room the same way as the carpet/pad.

HEPA vacuum the floor.

Leave air scrubber on, after removal, to help remove particulates. Move it in all directions and run machine for an hour for every 1600 cu. ft.

Go to the next room and repeat the process until all carpeted rooms have been completed.

Testing the rooms with a particle counter is an option to verify how much particulate matter may be left behind. It may be advisable to fog the rooms that need particle removal. Your IEP can make recommendations based on the particle test results.

CLEANING TECHNIQUES

BY CONTAMINATION LEVEL

Type of Contents	Condition 1 or 2 Known exposure	Condition 3 (Visible growth)
Porous Items	Photocopy or laminate to retain.	Photocopy or laminate to retain.
Paper		
Fabric	Launder using antimicrobial detergent such as borax and hot water, or dry clean (verify drycleaner's is in a non-contaminated building)	Likely must be disposed. Esporta washing machine (weighing the cost vs. value) may be an option.
Upholstered furniture	Cannot be cleaned	Cannot be cleaned
Mattress	Cannot be cleaned	Cannot be cleaned

Box springs	Cannot be cleaned	Cannot be cleaned
Unfinished wood,	HEPA vacuum/sand/apply anti-microbial/dry. Cold Fog with Concrobium "mold control", or "Aerosolver". Follow 2016 "CIRS consensus" document *(see appendix)* fogging instructions.	Dispose/replace if significantly rotten, or structurally damaged. HEPA vacuum/sand/apply CMSR (Concrobium Mold Stain Remover) using PPE (Personal Protective Equipment). Cold fog per 2016 "CIRS consensus" document *(see appendix)*
Unsealed ceramic	Cannot be cleaned	Cannot be cleaned
Non-Porous **Glass, Metal, Plastic, Sealed wood, etc.**	HEPA vacuum/wet wipe with anti-microbial/ dry. When dusting only, HEPA vacuum/dust using dry Swiffer cloth.	HEPA vacuum/scrubbing, immersion washing with ultrasonic bath, or steam cleaning/dry. Or HEPA vacuum/sanding and refinishing as applicable.

CONTENT CLEANING PROCEDURES CHECKLIST

Please read entire document first, before implementation. Ask questions to minimize misunderstanding(s). Any "no" responses to the questions below should be addressed with your IEP, prior to proceeding with any cleaning. Your IEP will be able to create a detailed cleaning plan to help ensure that the content cleaning process is done effectively and reduces the risk of cross contamination. This checklist will help with the organization of the cleaning work plan.

Client name:

_____

Site address:

_____

Date of Initial Walk Through:

_____

Walk Through Attended By:

_____

Remediation Completed: Yes/No

_____

Remediation Clearance Testing Pass: Yes/No

_____

Build Back Complete: Yes/ No

_____

Building science/home performance techniques completed? Yes/No

Remarks:

Do not remove contents from the rooms if remediation has not taken place. If remediation has not taken place start with **step one**. If remediation has taken place (or if no remediation is required and this is a "contents" and building cleaning process only), start with **stage one sort**. After stage one sort has been completed, proceed to stage two sort and stage three sort (these sorts can be done together or separately).

STEP ONE: Document contents with photographs and notes before moving contents. This will help to determine the extent of the exposure of the contents. Contents will be sorted by condition, then bagged and sealed using "goose neck" technique, or put into air-tight containers. Outsides of containers/bags will be wiped down with an approved anti- microbial (CIRS tolerable) then HEPA vacuumed while in the "exit decon chamber." Containers and or bagged items will be labeled by condition and placed in stage one sort location for condition sorting. Sort contents by condition status and store contents in pre-established storage container such as pod container, storage facility, or isolated prepared garage etc.) When all contents have been removed from the remediation area, the remediation process can begin. (see remediation checklist)

STAGE ONE SORT: Sort contents by their condition as described below:
    CONDITION 1: May have exposure to mycotoxins, spores, not visible.
    CONDITION 2: Exposure to mycotoxins, spores, not visible.
    CONDITION 3: Visible mold and or source condition.

STAGE TWO SORT: Using the sort list located in the Appendix, all items not to be cleaned need to be contained and removed from the vicinity to prevent further contamination and cross contamination. For example, do not put items in indoor trash cans, waste baskets etc. Ensure double bagging and seal all boxes for haul off.

STAGE THREE SORT BY TYPE OF MATERIAL: See level of contamination and recommended cleaning techniques form located in the Appendix. Sort by type of material and cleaning technique.

AFTER STAGE THREE SORT:

Contaminated contents should be double bagged in black bags or cardboard boxes that identify that they are "dirty" or contaminated. Once the contents have been cleaned, they will be put in clear bags or clear clean plastic boxes and stored in a "designated clean area." **Cleaned Contents are not to be placed in the building before receiving final building cleaning clearance results and walkthrough.**

Correction/Comments:

_____

_____

_____

_____

Content "cleaning" preparation steps: There are several cleaning methods, depending on the type of material to be cleaned and the level of contamination. Generally, the cleaning process is HEPA vacuuming/wet wipe with approved (CIRS tolerable) anti-microbial, then dry or allow to dry.

STEP ONE:

DEVELOP CLEANING ROOM/AREA: This can be a pre-cleaned garage with critical barriers that do not communicate with the building or another pod. A last resort would be a room within the building that is cleaned, with critical barriers (6 mil poly minimum), and controls in place (controls are tacky mats, sealed zipper doors, and "s" doors).

WHAT CONSTITUTES A CLEANING ROOM:

☐ Room ventilation (i.e. open window). If the outside is dusty or has pollens/particulates, then use tackified filters in the windows)

☐ Isolate doorways/critical barriers

☐ Tacky mats before entry

☐ Positive pressure in clean room

☐ Air scrubbers in clean room

☐ Down draft table

☐ Cleaning supplies

☐ Clear bags for clean contents

☐ Clear plastic air-tight storage boxes for cleaned contents

☐ HEPA vacuum

STEP TWO: CLEANING OPTIONS TO PICK FROM AS APPLICABLE

☐ HEPA vacuum, wet wipe, dry

☐ Air washing (leaf blower, fan)

☐ Power washing

☐ Steam (230-240 degrees)

☐ Chemical (shock wave by fiber lock) – the client must have been tolerance tested

☐ Esporta machine with certified operator (if available)

☐ Specialized laundry (drycleaners) verify chemical processes and confirm building is not water damaged.

STEP THREE: ORGANIZE CONTENT CLEANING PROCESS

☐ Sort contents by cleaning option

☐ Have a system for each step

☐ Isolate clean from dirty (people, items, equipment, supplies)

☐ Avoid cross contamination of secure areas and pathways

☐ Use clear or white clean bags for cleaned contents or clear plastic storage tubs for cleaned contents. this will help to identify clean contents more easily.

STEP FOUR: INITIATE POST CLEANING INSPECTION (WHITE GLOVE TEST, VISUAL TEST, AND SELECTED TESTING OF CONTENTS*)

☐ Content test methods

☐ Tape lift test

☐ Microvac test air test

---

*NOTE: Before cleaning all of your contents, it is critically important that you confirm that your cleaning process is working. To verify that your process is working and achieving the desired results, we suggest that you sample three times for each process, for each type of material. Testing should include three phases of testing on each different material. Phase one should be the white glove test. Phase two should be the visual test, and phase three should be either the tape lift test or microvac test, depending on the type of material being tested.

In most cases, if the process is successful on the test items, it should work well for the duration of the cleaning. However, **introducing new people, methods, or equipment can create breaches in the process.** If changes occur re-testing may be warranted. Unique surfaces or hard to clean items may need specific testing on that item.

Content test results

☐ PASS ☐ FAIL

REMARKS:

_____

_____

If contents pass the testing, contents may be brought into the building if IEP gives approval or the building has been tested to be clean.

If contents fail the testing, review the test results with your IEP and follow the IEP's recommendations.

Review how the clean room was set up, the process that was followed to clean the items and go back to step one or two depending on your findings. **In some cases, particular items may simply need to be discarded if they cannot be cleared via testing.**

REMARKS:

_____

_____

CONTENT SORT CHECKLIST

This checklist is used to simplify the sorting process. Before sorting your items, review "Contamination Conditions and Recommended Cleaning Techniques" in Appendix. That document will outline what will be involved in cleaning each item you choose to keep. Please note that if an item is **porous,** especially if it has tested positive for contamination, it may be impossible to clean adequately. If the item is considered personally sentimental or highly valuable, it should be put into a sealed container and stored for the time being. This period of extreme stress is not the best time to make these difficult decisions. When some time has passed and your health has improved, you will have the necessary perspective to decide the best way to deal with these items.

ITEMS TO GET RID OF:

☐ Throw away

☐ Sell

☐ Donate

ITEMS TO BE CLEANED BY A REMEDIATION COMPANY COMPLIANT WITH CIRS STANDARDS:

☐ Items to be cleaned in a containment area. (i.e. piano, etc.)

☐ Items to be cleaned by remediation company "soft". (i.e. Leather couch, etc.)

☐ Items to be cleaned by remediation company "hard". (i.e. dresser, TV, computers, etc.)

ITEMS HOMEOWNER WILL CLEAN:

☐ Items to be contained in sealed labeled containers to be cleaned at a future date.

☐ Items to be washed in a dishwasher.

☐ Items to be washed in a washing machine.

☐ Items to be washed via dipping and cleaning that are fragile.

☐ Items to be cleaned through the HEPA vacuum/wet wiping/down draft table/ air scrub cleaning process.

☐ Items that you're not sure what to do with, identify and ask IEP for recommendations.

ENDPOINT CRITERIA

Knowing your endpoint criteria is critical for successful remediation, building and content cleaning. Please see the endpoint criteria below:

1 – VISUAL INSPECTION

Were the specifications followed? Was the moisture source identified and corrected? Were the contents and debris removed? Was all visible mold removed? Was the work area white-glove dust free?

2 – TOTAL SPORE CONCENTRATION

Is the total spore concentration less than 2,000 c/m3 (typical of a normal fungal ecology)? If less than 800, go to criterion 4.

3 - COMPARISON TO MAKE UP AIR SOURCE

Is the total spore concentration of fungal material on the work area sample below that on the comparison sample?

Comparison sample collected from out-of-doors or inside building, but outside work area, depending on location of containment entry point.

4 - RANK / ORDER COMPARISON

Is the level of each fungal type (and hyphae) recovered from the work area less than 100 c/m3 above the level of the same fungal type (and hyphae) on the comparison sample?

5 - INDICATOR ORGANISMS

Were *Aspergillus/Penicillium*-like spores on the work area sample less than 200 c/m3?

6 – TARGET ORGANISMS

Was the work area sample free of target fungal types, both counted and observed?

Zero tolerance of Stachybotrys sp., Fusarium sp., Trichoderma sp., Memnoniella sp., Chaetomium sp.

Pinto, Michael. (2004). Mold clean-up projects: Post remediation criteria are critical to success. Professional Safety. Nov. 2004.

NOTE: Direct read samples must be examined with 1000x microscopy.

This endpoint criteria has been an extremely valuable tool for individuals with CIRS. It has been our direct experience that, without adhering to this criteria, anything less rigorous will not be adequate to support recovery.

HOME PERFORMANCE ASSESSMENT CHECKLIST

This check list will be used to identify specific measures of building science techniques known in the building industry as a *Home Performance Assessment.* A certified B.P.I (Building Performance Institute) professional with a building analyst certification can assess, test, and recommend specific home performance techniques.

Optimizing home performance can minimize cross contamination in the home, reduce toxin infiltration, create fresh air circulation, and reduce energy costs. **Implementation of these building performance techniques can often be the difference between success and failure for CIRS individuals and families.** Please review this checklist with your IEP and building performance professional as a guide to customize a plan for your "Healthy Home".

SITE CONCERNS: (See visual assessment checklist in Appendix)

_____

_____

EXTERIOR BUILDING CONCERNS: (See visual assessment checklist in Appendix).

_____

_____

GAS LEAK TESTING: The B.P.I. building analyst is certified to test accessible gas lines, fittings, and gas appliances, including gas meter or propane tank as applicable, using a gas leak detector.

The testing should include date stamped photographs of all noted gas leaks.

All discovered gas leaks are to be "verified" using a soap test bubble solution with supporting photographs.

Notify GSR (Gas Service Representative) if leaks cannot be repaired at the point of discovery.

If GSR is not available, all gas leaks, if not corrected during investigation, will need to be isolated and gas shut down until the repairs can be made. Note all outdated flex supply and shut off valves for replacement.

INFRARED (IR)

An IR camera is used during a home performance assessment. This tool helps to identify air infiltration, cross contamination issues, and will show vapor drive and other moisture conditions within the walls, or attic spaces.

Combustion Safety Testing
Combustion Appliance Zone (CAZ)

The combustion appliance zone (CAZ) is the area or areas within the home that contain gas fired appliance(s). It is important to identify and test the CAZ, to understand how the appliances are working (or not) in their respective CAZ areas. For example, combustion appliances that share the same space can have negative effects on each other. Larger appliances, such as a furnace, can create negative pressure within the space, causing the water heater, located in the same space, to back draft or malfunction. Sometimes the gas dryer, water heater, and furnace are all within the same space, which depending on the size of the space, can add to the safety hazard potential. Without testing the CAZ, there may be undetected malfunctions including large amounts of negative air pressure. This can create or exacerbate cross contamination as well as indoor air quality issues.

Dangerous levels of carbon monoxide may also exist. Systematic testing of each appliance individually first, then simultaneously, can detect malfunctions that you may not be aware of otherwise. **Combustion appliances can be one of the most prevalent sources of indoor air pollution if they are not operating correctly. They are capable of adding CO (carbon monoxide), and high particulate counts due to poor combustion.**

It is vital to perform a combustion safety test on all combustion appliances including gas furnaces, water heaters, gas fireplaces, gas dryers, and gas stoves. Combustion safety testing will ensure that the appliance has been installed correctly, is operating safely, and that there are no gas leaks, or CO (Carbon monoxide) problems during combustion. It is important to note that putting the house in a negative pressure "worst case" condition, to test the appliances, can sometimes cross contaminate the home. Potential toxins may be pulled into the home while the home is in this negative pressurized testing state.

It is important to know that some sensitized CIRS individuals may react to the negative pressures that will be set up (by turning on existing exhaust fans, exhaust hoods, and dryers). It is advisable to discuss the potential reaction and evaluate the risk based on the individual. It may be that this test is performed when the individual is not present. A plan may need to be put in place to air scrub, using a diffuser tail, after the test to minimize adverse health effects. (See Appendix)

All combustion safety concerns that arise during the combustion safety testing will be noted and corrected as per the B.P.I standards, in conjunction with the overall sequenced work plan. To ensure health, life safety issues will be given highest priority.

Carbon Monoxide Testing

Ambient CO levels shall be monitored upon entering the combustion appliance zone and during the test period of all of the appliances. Both vented (water heater), and unvented (range) appliances will be tested using B.P.I. professional standards for specific procedures and thresholds.

Worst Case Condition and Depressurization

As stated above, worst-case depressurization represents the most negative pressure condition that can be created in the home. There are worst case depressurization limit tables for the appliances. Knowing what the worst case depressurization is in the home, and how the combustion appliances may be affected, will help to identify and correct any adverse conditions such as gas leaks, and CO poisoning.

Duct Testing NOTE: CIRS INDIVIDUALS MAY HAVE SEVERE REACTIONS TO HIGH VOLUMES OF AIR PRESSURE CHANGES. IT IS NOT RECOMMENDED TO PERFORM A BLOWER DOOR TEST NOR A DLTO (DUCT LEAKAGE TO OUTSIDE TEST) USING A BLOWER DOOR, EVEN IF USING POSITIVE PRESSURE. CAUSING PRESSURE CHANGES IN THE HOME CAN EXACERBATE SYMPTOMS FOR THE CIRS INDIVIDUAL. It is recommended to perform a total duct leakage test with cleaned equipment to obtain duct leakage results so as not to create too much indoor pressure change.

If the home has a ducted furnace or HVAC (Heating, Ventilation, and Air Conditioning) system, this system can be tested by pressurizing the ducting system itself and calculating how much duct leakage the system has. The average duct leakage in California is 30%. Most of this leakage is due to the fact that most systems built before 2015 may have been "sealed" using "duct tape" which typically degrades over time (especially in a hot attic). This allows the ducting system to leak. This leak can be a source for toxins and particulates as the system pulls air from these undesirable areas such as crawlspaces, attics, or within wall cavities.

If your home was built before the 1978, it should be inspected for other potential toxins and health hazards such as asbestos building materials, asbestos-wrapped ducting, fiberglass furnace ducting, and lead based paint. If asbestos wrapped ducting is identified to be part of the ducting system, the ducting system should not be tested. Asbestos wrapped ducting is considered a potential health hazard and should be removed by a licensed asbestos abatement contractor, using best practices for removal to avoid contaminating the home.

In some states of the US, there are "energy efficiency" programs offered by utility companies. These offer rebate incentives for making a home more energy efficient. The energy upgrade programs identify air sealing and duct sealing as two important ways to improve air quality while also reducing energy losses. For those that live in an area with these programs available, it might make financial sense to investigate these utility cash incentives to help offset the cost of the upgrades. There are also "Green Energy" loans that have attractive rates to help provide financial assistance for the energy upgrades.

How much air do I need?

We need generally a minimum of one third of the total volume of air in a home to be exchanged for fresh air every hour. As humans, we generate up to 3 quarts of water vapor a day, expelling the vapors from our mouth. We also create vapors and moisture by using the shower, dryer, dishwasher, and stove. The vapor and moisture, along with the combustion appliances in a home, can give off VOC's and other particulates. As one third of the volume of the home's air must come from a fresh air source per hour, it is recommended to install an HRV (Heat recovery ventilator) or ERV (energy recovery Ventilator), depending on the climate.

These air exchange machines are made to pull stale air out of specific areas of the home, such as kitchens or baths, and bring in fresh air into specific living areas of the home, such as bedrooms or living rooms. These units have a built-in heat exchanger that tempers the air as it travels by the heat exchanger, adjusting the air temperature within a few degrees of the conditioned space air.

For CIRS individuals, the HRV or ERV is a vital addition to a home. The ventilator system allows the complete air sealing of the home to prevent cross contamination. It provides the right amount of fresh air into the home

while pulling out the stale air, moisture, and vapors, keeping the indoor climate fresh and dry. The incoming air is also filtered to reduce pollens, and other irritants from coming into the home. Your IEP or B.P.I. analyst can recommend the right unit for your needs to be incorporated into the work plan.

HOUSE HUNTING

When looking for a new living space, it is important to narrow your search to those environments that are least likely to have mold toxin problems:

1. Choose newer built structures that are not older than 8 years, or 10 years if well maintained. They are less likely to have sustained water damage if they have been well built and well maintained in this time frame. However, age alone does not exclude this possibility.

2. Avoid flat roof designs or multiple roof lines/angles as they are notorious for having problems. Water intrusion is more likely due to standing water and roof line integrity problems.

3. Examine under and around sinks, refrigerator, dishwasher, washer/dryer, toilets, tubs, showers and water heater areas for obvious signs of water damage. Even old water stains can be significant. Inspect ceilings of closets for mold and note any "musty" smells.

4. Note if there is an exterior irrigation or sprinkler system that leaves water pooling next to home, or sprays water on wood trim, siding, wood decks, entries etc. Landscaping should be graded away from the house.

5. Avoid raised floor crawlspaces and structures with subterranean rooms, such as homes built into hillsides. Avoid structures with leaky basements or areas that may be exposed to flood or water intrusion damage (currently or in the past).

6. Confirm that there is adequate attic ventilation and if an air conditioner is located in the attic, confirm that the drain pan for the evaporator coil is intact and that it drains appropriately to the outside.

7. Avoid carpet, if at all possible, to avoid a potential "reservoir of contaminates".

8. Ask if any known water damage has occurred, not if they have mold. If the answer is yes, it is not for you. Many people find themselves back in an unsafe environment because they have not been able to screen well enough initially.

Narrow down your choices based on this information to the best of your ability.

The next step is to collect dust from areas of the home as directed by Mycometrics Laboratory. They will send you a kit with a "swiffer" cloth and complete instructions. (See Resources for contact information and Appendix for a sample letter explaining to the landlord or seller why this test is necessary.)

This test is called an ERMI (Environmental Relative Moldy Index) test. The dust sample will be analyzed, by the lab, for mold DNA. The test results are sent back to you and can be evaluated by your IEP or your certified practitioner. This is one valuable tool for assessing the potential health impact of a specific indoor environment.

Once you have narrowed down your selection, arrange to spend several hours, or overnight in the space to be certain that you do not react to other potential contaminants (VOC's, MVOC's, etc.)

The extra time and effort invested during this process will pay off in huge dividends. Choosing potential living spaces carefully will save time, money, frustration and potentially devastating health consequences down the road.

HOUSEHOLD PROACTIVE MAINTENANCE CHECKLIST

Plumbing fixtures (check daily): toilets, under all sinks, showers, clothes washer, dish washer, refrigerators and automatic ice makers, and hot water heaters. Any indication of water leaking from these areas needs to be addressed immediately.

Any fans that are installed to eliminate moisture, such as in bathrooms and laundry rooms, need to be functioning correctly.

Periodic checks need to be scheduled for furnace, air conditioning units, attic and crawlspace areas.

HVAC filters need to be changed on a regular basis.

All windows and doors need to be routinely inspected for problems with possible leaks or problems with sealing.

Flooring needs to be routinely inspected for moisture problems (i.e. bubbling rippling or buckling.)

Periodic duct work inspection and cleaning needs to be scheduled.

Check all roof penetrations and general condition of roofing components, such as chimney flashing, roof to wall metal, plumbing vents, flashing, and skylights.

Make sure all penetrations are well sealed. Inspect fascia and roof overhang materials to ensure the materials are not degrading, cracked, or peeling.

Ongoing rigorous cleaning efforts include:

- Weekly HEPA vacuuming of floors and sofas.
- Weekly dusting of surfaces with microfiber cloths.
- Weekly wet mop floors
- Avoid clutter!

Once or twice yearly:

Whole house cleaning or fogging depending on amount of activity going on in the home.

NOTE: Be certain that "sewer/water backup" is included in your homeowner's insurance policy. This event is often NOT covered, and can be financially catastrophic for an individual with CIRS.

INITIAL CLIENT INTAKE FORM

Initial Client Intake Form

Name:		Date:	

Address:

Phone #:		City/State/zip:	

Email:

Diagnosis:

Doctor:		Office Phone#:	

Symptoms:

HEALTH HISTORY:

Date: Mo/Yr

Time line

When did health begin to decline?

Was there a triggering event?

Have you done any medical tests such as VCS, HLA, Neuroquant, nasal culture, etc? If so, please list?

Number of people in household?

Does anyone else in the household have similar symptoms?

Who:	Relation:	Age:
Who:	Relation:	Age:

What treatments have you undergone?

Are you taking any additional supplements? If so, what?

If you work, what is your profession?

What type of establishment do you work? Office, restaurant, etc..

Do you work outdoors? ☐ Yes ☐ No

What type of work do the other members of the household do?

HOME HISTORY:

Residence:

☐ House	☐ Duplex	☐ Rent
☐ Condo	☐ Apartment	☐ Own

Setting:

☐ Rural	☐ Sub division
☐ Urban	☐ Water front

Year Built: _____ **Year Purchased:** _____

Plans Available? ☐ Yes ☐ No

Square footage: _____ How long at this residence? _____

Attached Garage: ☐ Yes ☐ No

Foundation Type: ☐ Slab ☐ Raised

Type of heating? ☐ Forced Air ☐ Wall furnace ☐ Space ☐ Fire place

Location? ☐ Attic ☐ Crawl space ☐ Garage ☐ Interior Closet

Fuel type? ☐ Nat Gas ☐ Electric ☐ Propane ☐ Wood

Ductwork present? ☐ Yes ☐ No

Location? ☐ Attic ☐ Crawl space ☐ Between floors

Have any water events occurred to your knowledge? Please explain with dates, who did the work and how it was remediated.

Event 1: _____
_____
_____

Event 2: _____
_____
_____

Event 3: _____
_____
_____

Is there visible mold now? ☐ Yes ☐ No

Where? _____

Do you smell mold? ☐ Yes ☐ No

Where? _____

What rooms do you feel worse in? _____

What rooms do you feel better in? _____

Have there been any additions or remodels to your knowledge?
Please explain with dates, who did the work and what was included as part of the project.

Remodel 1: _____
_____
_____

Remodel 2: _____
_____
_____

If you have any test results such as ERMI, HERTSMI-2, Air/ tape samples, etc...
Please attach them as digital copies with this form to:

REBUILDING CHECKLIST

This rebuild check list may be used to review with the IEP, Remediation Company, or contractor. This checklist is designed to implement specific scopes of work after your remediation has been completed to the point of rebuilding your home and for new build considerations. All applicable checklist items must be considered and implemented to minimize mold growth, reduce cross contamination, prevent future water intrusion, and improve the overall indoor air quality of the home.

This checklist has the PRE-REQUISITE that all water events, and moisture intrusion events have been corrected, mold has been properly remediated, controls are still in place (such as isolation barriers from other parts of the home), supply and return duct registers are still sealed, and all exterior site conditions have been addressed, that may be a contributing factor to the water damage to the home. This checklist's primary focus relates to building back for the building interior.

Air seal: Combustion safety testing should always be performed before air sealing. (See home performance in Appendix). Seal wall-framing plates at the bottom of a wall (between the concrete slab or the wood sub floor) and at the top of a wall (at the attic plane), to prevent air from the wall cavities from infiltrating into the conditioned space (interior living space) of the home. Air seal all wall, floor, and ceiling plane penetrations (such as plumbing and electrical penetrations) to prevent cross contamination.

Attic venting: Attic venting may also include solar roof vents, and or gable end vents that use temperature and humidistat controls.

Baseboard: Do not use MDF (multi density fiberboard). Use pine or other solid wood products, but apply zero VOC primers on all sides and at all joints. Use zero/low VOC stains and clear finishes that are well tolerated by the CIRS patient. Install baseboard on clear rubber bumpers and install base shoe to hide the elevated base.

Cabinets: Use zero VOC cabinet finishes Use plywood cores, not chip board or particle board cabinets. Base cabinets should be made to be suspended above the floor using waterproof legs, or ¼" bumpers to elevate the cabinets. Include removable toe kicks. In the case of a water event, the toe kicks can be removed and accessibility can be maintained to remove water under the cabinets.

Caulking/Paints: If chemical sensitivities are an issue, use zero VOC caulking and paints to reduce indoor VOC levels.

Electrical: Use foam gaskets behind all electrical receptacles, and switch cover plates. Seal these to the wall using zero VOC caulking to prevent air leaks and cross contamination. Perform combustion safety testing before applying this recommendation, if applicable. (See Home Performance checklist)

Exhaust fans: Exhaust fans must be vented to the outside, not in the floor or attic space, as that will invite mold growth and rodents. In wet areas, such as bathrooms, laundry rooms, exhaust fans should include a moisture sensor built into the fan which will operate the fan automatically when the moisture is detected by the fan sensor. If you have an existing fan that does not have an automatic moisture sensor, you can simply install a "Dew stop" moisture detection switch, if it is in the same room as the fan. This will allow the fan to operate to remove vapor and moisture from the home, without having to remember to turn it on or off.

It is important to install an exhaust fan even if you have a window in a bathroom or laundry room. Many people do not open a window routinely, and the window does not remove the moisture as well as an exhaust fan that is positioned well, and is of the right size for the room. We have seen many showers with windows that have moldy ceilings. Often, exhaust fans are installed using the minimum size and quality. Attention to proper size of the fan, and features, such as a moisture sensor, is critical. And as always, exhaust fans must be ducted to the outside of a building to prevent moisture, and mold damage.

Exterior surfaces: Ensure that an effective vapor barrier, that eliminates vapor drive, moisture, and wind, is used as a means of protecting the outside walls of the home.

One example would be a building wrap product such as "Dupont" brand Tyvek "Home Wrap" which is designed to help keep air and water out, while letting water vapor escape. For doors and windows, using "flex wrap" door and window flashings will ensure that all penetrations and junctions, where dissimilar materials meet, are fully water proofed. There are many products that are available to eliminate moisture and vapor drive issues for a variety of home substrates and conditions.

Flooring: It is recommended to use zero VOC flooring such as hardwood, linoleum, bamboo, cork, etc. Avoid wall-to-wall carpeting. Carpeting can become a "reservoir" of contaminates and can be very high maintenance to keep clean enough for a CIRS individual. Remember to use low or zero VOC glues if glues are required for installation. Use small rugs that can be rolled up and removed to be cleaned in a commercial or offsite facility.

Foundations: Drainage is critical to be sloped away from the house at a minimum of 2% grade. Install a rock layer of 6", with a layer of 15 mil vapor barrier such as "Stego wrap" over the rock layer, using "Beastfoot" form staking method to prevent penetrations in the vapor barrier. Any such penetration can result in water intrusion. French drains around perimeter of the footings should be in operation to remove all subterranean water from the foundation and away from the building foundations or basement. Eliminate planters and planting against the building.

Garages: Garage slabs need to have concrete curbs and floors that slope toward the exterior door. The garage doors should have a watertight seal and sloped to drain away from the garage. Garage walls and ceilings should be finished. Exposed rough framing is nearly impossible to keep clean enough, if the framing is left exposed.

HVAC: Avoid HVAC systems that use ducting to distribute heating and cooling. Ductless mini split HVAC devices will avoid ducting altogether, preventing duct cross contamination, cleaning and maintenance challenges. Mini split systems are very energy efficient and can be installed in a variety of climate zones. If the mini split is not an option, and you must install a ducted system, use galvanized sheet metal in lieu of flex ducting. Seal the ducted system using ASTM rated 181 tape. The system should not leak more than 2%. Install a drain pan under the unit that is piped to the outside. Add a sensor that will shut down the system if water dumps into the pan. All supply boots must be sealed to prevent air leakage as well as return air plenums. Do not use fiberglass "duct board" on the inside of the plenum it should be installed on the outside to insulate the plenum.

Insulation: Use dense packed insulation for exterior walls. This material will not allow air to pass through the wall cavity as easily as insulation batts, and it offers a higher energy efficiency. Depending on exposure tests, one may use blown in cellulose, or fiberglass. Remember to dehumidify the insulation before installing wallboard to prevent trapped moisture from the dense packing. Attic insulation should only be installed after air sealing the attic plane, to minimize cross contamination and improve energy efficiency.

Metal Framing: Metal framing is preferable to wood framing.

Roof: Use plywood for the roof sheathing that includes a radiant barrier. OSB (Oriented Stranded Board) is not recommended because it molds significantly faster than plywood when water or moisture is present. The difference in cost is minimal. Ensure that the roof has sufficient venting, both high and low, to create proper airflow in the attic. This will help to prevent early breakdown of roofing materials, and moisture in the attic from condensation. Do not install dense packed insulation in cathedral or flat roofs. This will cause condensation, and mold growth, within the roof cavity. Ensure all roof penetrations have the correct flashings, are properly sealed, and use proper drip edge metals. Install ice shield on roof, valley's, and eaves, extending up past exterior wall lines two feet, as region dictates. Ensure that all roof to wall and chimney flashings are methodically and correctly installed.

Plumbing: Install shut off valves (angle stops) at each sink, dishwasher appliance, and toilet. Plan, if possible, to have accessible service areas where water can be turned off and on using isolation valves for quick response and viewing, especially for tub drains and valves. The washing machine drain hose should be fastened into the plumbing drain, not simply resting loose in it. The vibration from the washing machine can vibrate the drain hose allowing water to drain onto the floor.

Tank water heaters should have their T&P (temperature and Pressure) line piped to the outside. Tank water heaters should have a "Smitty pan" under the water heater that is piped to the outdoors. In case of a water heater leak, the water will drain to the outside of the home instead of inside. All supply hoses or flexible connections are to be braided stainless hoses for all plumbing fixtures such as washing machines, toilets, sinks dishwashers, etc. Floor drains should be installed in laundry and or tanked water heater areas to collect water overflows.

Shower/tub walls: For a backer board for framing showers, tub walls/ceiling use a water-resistant product such as "Dens Shield tile backer" under water proofing lath and plaster substrate. All shower pans should be leak tested for 24 hrs. to ensure the shower pan liner does not leak. Shower pan liners should be installed on a pre-sloped floor to allow proper drainage into the drain weep holes of the shower drain.

Trim/baseboard: Avoid using MDF (Medium Density Board) where there can be moisture, or high humidity. MDF typically can mold behind the baseboard once humidity or moisture is present. It also swells and, once exposed to water, swells and degrades quickly. Interior baseboard should be made of solid pine or hardwood, prefinished on all sides and installed with bumpers to elevate the baseboard from direct water immersion.

Wall surfaces: For interior wall surfaces, basements, or high moisture areas, use moisture and water resistant wallboard such as "Dens Armor plus" made by Georgia Pacific in lieu of standard gypsum drywall. This will give you added mold and moisture protection. It is important to follow the recommended paint/priming application instructions for additional mold resistance and wall protection.

Windows: Windows should be installed with the correct flashing, optimally double paned insulated units that do not create condensation. Window tracks should be kept clean and the weep holes, located at the bottom sill, should be free of obstructions to allow drainage. This includes patio doors as well.

Wood Framing: Check lumber for mold before installation, even if it is "new". Apply a mold growth inhibitor as protection against future water damage events, or excessive moisture problems. "Mold Control", made by Concrobium, is one such product that can be used on exposed framing members. Follow manufactures recommendations and allow to dry thoroughly. This product will inhibit future mold growth and is nontoxic. Exposure testing should always be done to verify patient compatibility. Test moisture content of wood framing before applying substrates, such as wallboard, to ensure dryness. Again, avoid using OSB (Oriented Stranded Board). OSB molds significantly faster than plywood when water or moisture is present.

REMEDIATION CHECKLIST

This checklist may be used to review with the IEP or Remediation Company to ensure that specific details are considered and included, as applicable, for your specific remediation process. All applicable check list items must be incorporated in the work plan with written procedural instructions, prior to implementation for optimal results. A jobsite meeting with personnel, prior to job start, to review each aspect of the processes will help to reveal breaches in the work processes and avoid misunderstandings prior to implementation.

Client name:

_____

Site address:

_____

Date of water event:

_____

Date of discovery of water event:

_____

The following must be included in the development of the work plan:

Verify the endpoint goals (see endpoint criteria for CIRS in Appendix). For the CIRS individual, the endpoint goals for CIRS must be met to be successful. All parties involved must follow the written CIRS work plan as a minimum standard. Working to a lower standard will prevent recovery for CIRS individuals. It is critical that the persons that are performing the work, including the post

remediation testing, have reviewed, understand, and agree to follow these processes within the work plan and endpoint criteria for CIRS.

☐ Pre-approve all cleaners, anti-microbial, fungicides, remediation products and materials to be used during process with owner before use. CIRS individual may need to perform exposure test verify product compatibility.

☐ Sketch/site diagram of decontamination unit, critical barriers, negative air machines, (NAM), material to be removed, waste to be generated and location of waste container onsite for disposal, materials and equipment to be staged.

☐ Contaminate source(s), location and type of contaminate.

☐ Hazard check (electrical, water, gas, debris, demolition, tools, equipment, etc.)

☐ Entry, pathways, and exit points

☐ Work zone(s)

☐ Bathroom facilities/protocol for use

☐ Monitor relative humidity (to be kept below 60%)

☐ Furnace and or HVAC system must be turned off. Plan to use alternate or temporary heating and cooling sources.

All supply and return duct grilles are to be sealed off (isolation barriers) and unit is turned off, to minimize cross contamination.

Mechanical systems to be checked and tested for contaminates.

Duct systems should be tested for "Total duct leakage" using the total duct leakage to outside measurement.

Warning: Do not use the "DLTO" (duct leakage to outside) test method. Using a blower door for a CIRS client can cause a catastrophic health reaction, even when using positive blower door pressure for testing.

- Plan for "contents" in work areas to be transported out of work area.
- Designated location for contaminated contents to be stored.

All equipment to be pre-cleaned by a three-step process

1. HEPA vacuum
2. Anti-microbial wet wiped including the wheels, cords, etc.
3. Allow equipment to dry. (This will avoid cross contamination)

☐ PPE (personal protective equipment)

☐ Containment(s), size

☐ Decontamination chamber

☐ Size isolation barriers

☐ Minimum negative pressures in remediation work zones.

☐ Exhaust negative air machines to out of doors.

☐ If windows in work areas are required to be open, install open window vents with tackified filters.

☐ Place tacky mats with removable sheets in work areas at entry and exit points.

☐ Work practices, including HEPA vacuum attachments to power tools, to minimize dust.

☐ Bag waste as work progresses (clean as you go policy enforced).

☐ Double bag for exiting containment (i.e. HEPA vacuum/wet wipe bag with approved anti-microbial).

☐ Small particle remediation must be performed once remediation has been completed but before mold testing. Use approved CIRS tolerable products and consensus document instructions. (See consensus document link in Resources).

Do not remove containment or barriers until all of the following has been verified. Some situations mandate that rooms that have been decontaminated must be kept in isolation until the whole house has been through a small particle cleaning. This precaution is to prevent cross contamination.

1. Endpoint criteria has been met and approved by IEP/client.

2. Build back work plan has been created and approved by IEP/client.

3. Written and approval from IEP/owner has been given upon the sign off-of the above two items.

By signing below, I have read, understood, and will implement these procedures.

IEP Print Name:

_____

Signature: _____ Date: _____

Client Print Name:

_____

Signature: _____ Date: _____

Remediation Contractor Name:

_____

Signature: _____ Date: _____

TEST DAY

WHAT TO EXPECT

CIRS CLIENTS, Please read and initial test day protocol items.

TEST DAY PROTOCOL

_____Please do not use wood burning fireplaces the day before the assessment, and we ask that the ashes are removed 24 hours before test day.

_____The infrared camera is best used with a high temperature difference between indoors/outdoors, so we like to start testing at 8:30 a.m.

_____As we will need full access to all parts of the home including the garage, attic, utility closets, attic, crawl spaces, under sinks, all rooms of the home, please make sure pathways are clear and unobstructed.

_____We will be moving air through your home, via your exhaust fans, dryers, etc. Please close all exterior windows and open all interior doorways.

_____Upon arrival, please let us know which bathroom is available for our use.

_____Full access and control of all appliances, including water heaters and furnaces will be required as we test. Please refrain from showering, cooking, laundry or using the appliances during the test period.

_____Combustion safety testing will be performed on all combustions appliances, and accessible gas or propane lines during the pre-and post-testing to ensure your safety and ours. All immediate safety concerns will be addressed upon discovery.

_____All pets must be contained away from operating equipment for safety. Household Birds must be kept in their cages during the full assessment period.

If you have any further questions or concerns, please feel free to contact me to discuss. We look forward to working with you!

VISUAL BUILDING
ASSESSMENT CHECKLIST

This checklist, along with the ERMI/HERTSMI-2 scoring result, is an essential tool to determine a safe environment. Include date stamped photographs for reference documentation.

Client name:

_____

Site address:

_____

Date of assessment:

_____

Year home was originally built:

_____

Year(s) remodeled:

_____

Areas remodeled:

_____

Create site map (such as Google map) of lot showing location of residence(s) and all buildings including orientation (north arrow), trees, water features including hot tubs, pools, creeks, site drainage, area drains, and septic tanks and or leach fields.

Create overlay of topography of site and adjoining properties to evaluate water shed, and topography both natural and manmade.

Exterior assessment: Noting the site maps above, walk around the exterior of the home and out buildings noting: Outside temperature/time of day _____ / _____

Outside humidity time of day _____ / _____

Indoor humidity time of day _____ / _____

Identify moisture issues

☐ Drainage systems

☐ Drainage outlets

☐ Drainage inlets

☐ Gutters/downspouts

☐ Water shed paths of travel

☐ Ponds

☐ Swimming pool

☐ Roof leaks/skylights/condition/installation

☐ Condensation

☐ Vegetation against the house or out buildings

☐ Peeling paint

Structural issues

☐ Roof sags

☐ Fascia/ overhang dry rot

☐ Rotten wood/trim

☐ Cracks in structure

Miscellaneous exterior

☐ Fire wood against or near the house

☐ Fences, gates

☐ Mulch, bark, against or near the house

☐ Manure, chicken pens, animal feces, hay near the house.

☐ Garbage, trash piles

☐ Exterior stucco/ is weep screed installed above the finish surface to allow moisture to drain from the stucco?

Health safety issues (exterior)

☐ Electrical

☐ Asbestos

☐ Visible mold

☐ Visible mildew

☐ Trip hazards

☐ Lead based paints

☐ Chemicals

Exterior wall penetrations

☐ Venting

☐ Plumbing

☐ Fans

☐ Doors

HVAC equipment

☐ Heat pump

☐ Swamp cooler

☐ Mini-split

☐ Furnace

Verify in operation

☐ CO monitor on each floor (low level type)

☐ Smoke detectors in each bedroom and on each floor.

Windows/skylights

☐ Type

☐ Condition

☐ Installation

☐ Size

Crawlspace:

Under-floor crawlspaces should be typically assessed as the last part of the assessment so that the investigator can put on PPE (personal protective equipment) consisting of a Tyvek suit (booties, and attached hood, gloves, respirator, safety glasses). The investigator should inspect the crawl space from an outside access, then remove the suit outdoors and leave it to minimize the exposure to the CIRS individual and their home.

If the only crawlspace access is inside the home, setting up a containment surrounding the opening and using negative air pressure to the crawlspace during the investigation will minimize contamination. Remove the PPE as you come back into the containment, put the PPE into a sealed bag, wipe down the containment, and HEPA vacuum the bag and floor surfaces to minimize cross contamination.

☐ Size, quantity and condition of crawlspace venting (determine minimum venting requirements as per local building code)

☐ Floor plane penetrations

☐ Insulation/ type

☐ Moisture issues soil

☐ Mold

☐ Rot

☐ Standing water

☐ Moisture issues plumbing leaks/type

☐ Drainage issues

☐ Vapor barrier

☐ Fans/location/direction/size

☐ Heating/HVAC ducting/type/condition

☐ Exposed electrical boxes, improper wiring, or connections

☐ Earth to wood contact or debris

☐ Open tub drain areas

☐ Rodent/animals

☐ Access door

☐ Tub access

Interior inspection/walk through

Smells (musty, moldy, dirt, feces)

_____

_____

Sensing (warm, cold, stuffy, humid, hot, moisture, dry, smoky)

_____

_____

Moisture issues

☐ Active leaks

☐ Visible moisture

☐ Visible mold

☐ Historical leaks

☐ Historical mold

☐ Vinyl floors discolored

☐ Paint peeling

☐ Ceiling stains

☐ Wood rot

☐ Moisture damage

☐ Wet materials

Hazards

☐ Asbestos

☐ Lead

☐ VOC's

☐ CO (carbon monoxide)

- [ ] Chemical contaminates
- [ ] Mold
- [ ] Garage connections to house
- [ ] Combustible materials
- [ ] Gas leaks

Exhaust fans

- [ ] Bath fans/verify venting to the outside
- [ ] Oven hoods/verify venting to the outside
- [ ] Whole house fans sealed or unsealed? Location?

Fireplaces: gas _____ wood _____ pellet _____

Windows: type _____ condition _____

Interior doors: type _____ condition _____

Wall penetrations
Ceiling penetrations

Lighting: sealed _____ unsealed _____

Duct registers: sealed _____ unsealed _____

Furnishings: (note all that has been exposed to water damage)

- [ ] Antique
- [ ] Furniture against walls
- [ ] Clothes/shoes in closet
- [ ] Toys

☐ Sofas

☐ Stove

☐ Water heater

☐ Furnace

☐ Gas fireplace

APPLIANCES (All combustion safety testing should be performed, on all gas fired appliances, by a professional certified to perform a combustion safety test such as a B.P.I (Building Performance Institute) professional with a building analyst certification. The combustion safety test will confirm that your gas fired appliances are operating safely. This is a "must do" before any air sealing occurs, to eliminate the possibility of a health hazard. CO (Carbon Monoxide) can be the by-product of poorly installed, old, or air restricted combustion appliances. **Never air seal without confirming that the combustion safety test has been executed, all failures, if any, have been corrected and the combustion safety re-test is verified to pass.**

DISCLAIMER

MEDICAL

This manual is NOT to be used as a "Do It Yourself" guide! Your journey to recovery requires partnering with an expert in CIRS. The instructions and checklists, contained in this Appendix, are to be followed with the guidance of your Certified CIRS Practitioner.

The Shoemaker Protocol is a scientific approach to successful treatment of CIRS. While the protocol is to be followed precisely, unique individual responses may require adjustment in the initial dosage of meds and speed of progression through the sequential steps of the protocol.

We strongly recommend that you partner with a Shoemaker Certified CIRS Practitioner for an accurate Diagnosis and Treatment Plan.

FACTS ABOUT CIRS

FOR FRIENDS & FAMILY

Chronic Inflammatory Response Syndrome (CIRS) is very REAL and diagnosed by specific blood tests, vision tests, and a cluster of predictable symptoms.

- 24 % of people have the gene that makes them susceptible to **CIRS**.
- The gene must be ACTIVATED for the immune system to be triggered.

Activation may be caused by infection, allergic reaction, pregnancy, surgery, severe physical or emotional trauma, or any event that results in acute inflammation.

Once the gene is activated, **every exposure to a water damaged building will make them sicker & sicker.**

Exposure to mold (dead or alive), mold fragments, mold by-products, and other inflammatory chemicals found in water damaged buildings, will cause the immune system to release inflammatory chemical into the circulation. Inhaling unseen mold toxins triggers massive inflammation in the body (including the brain) of someone with **CIRS.**

Mold does not need to be visible to cause harm to the individual with CIRS. Microscopic particles of mold toxins can be inhaled from heating or air conditioning ducts, carpets, upholstered furniture, and air drawn from within wall spaces in tightly sealed buildings.

48 hours of dampness from a minor leak or water intrusion is enough to make carpet, drywall, furniture and other porous surfaces a reservoir of mold, mold fragments, bacteria and mold toxins.

It is easy to discount the complaints of someone with CIRS because the environments that cause them severe symptoms have little or NO effect on those without the gene or in those who have not had their genetic profile activated.

The most common symptoms of CIRS include: Severe fatigue, headaches, light sensitivity, muscle & joint pain, tingling, numbness, difficulty concentrating, mood swings, decreased recent memory, dizziness, sinus congestion, abdominal pain, tremors and extreme thirst.

The individual with CIRS is strongly cautioned by his or her physician to AVOID EXPOSURE TO WATER DAMAGED BUILDINGS. Failure to follow this advice will make recovery impossible. PLEASE do not be offended if a friend or family member tells you they cannot visit your home, workplace or favorite restaurant. Their health depends on it!

HLA RESULT CORRELATIONS

	DRB1	DQ	DRB3	DRB4	DRB5
	4	3		53	
Multisusceptible	11/12	3	52B		
	14	5	52B		
	7	2/3		53	
Mold Susceptible	13	6	52A, B, C		
	17	2	52A		
	18*	4	52A		
Borrelia, post Lyme Syndrome	15	6			51
	16	5			51
Dinoflagellates	4	7/8		53	
Multiple Antibiotic Resistant Staph Epidermis (MARCoNS)	11	7	52B		
No recognized significance	8	3, 4, 6			
	7	9		53	
Low-risk Mold	12	7	52B		
	9	9		53	

From: Ritchie C. Shoemaker MD. Lab Tests. www.survivingmold.com

INITIAL CIRS DATA FORM

How long have you been suffering from Chronic Illness?

What year did your symptoms begin?

What was the progression of symptoms?

What diagnoses have you been given and when?

What lab tests or imaging studies have been done to validate the diagnoses and when?

What are your 6 most prominent symptoms currently?

_____

_____

Do you have any family members with similar symptoms?

Have you ever lived in a water-damaged building?

Have you experienced a tick bite? When?

Have you been in a high-risk situation for tick bites? When?

Have you ever traveled to a tropical locale? When?

Have you eaten or handled tropical reef fish such as barracuda, grouper, red snapper, eel, amberjack, sea bass or Spanish mackerel.

Have you lived in or traveled to an area affected by algae "blooms"?

When? _____ Where _____

Do you react adversely to scents, chemical smells, or smoke?

LIVING ENVIRONMENTS (Most Recent First)

Moved In	Left	Brief Description	Symptoms
_____	_____	_____	_____
_____	_____	_____	_____
_____	_____	_____	_____
_____	_____	_____	_____
_____	_____	_____	_____

WORK / SCHOOL ENVIRONMENTS (Most Recent First))

Started	Left	Brief Description	Symptoms
_____	_____	_____	_____
_____	_____	_____	_____
_____	_____	_____	_____
_____	_____	_____	_____

Other factors affecting health including surgeries, trauma, severe stress, NOT already listed (Most Recent First)

Date	Event
_____	_____
_____	_____
_____	_____
_____	_____
_____	_____

LAB RESULTS TRACKING FORM

NAME:

_____

DOB

_____

Date Diagnosed: _____ HLA: _____ _____

Environmental Consultation:

_____

ERMI: home _____ work _____

Labs:	MSH	VIP	C4a	TGFB1	MMP9	VEGF	VCS
Date:	___	___	___	___	___	___	___
	___	___	___	___	___	___	___
	___	___	___	___	___	___	___
	___	___	___	___	___	___	___
	___	___	___	___	___	___	___

MARCONS Culture: Date/ + or - (circle)

_____ + - _____ + - _____ + - _____ + - _____ + -

ERMI/HERTSMI-2: Date & Result

_____ / _____   _____ / _____   _____ / _____   _____ / _____

LAB SPECIMEN OPTIONS

*Additional information on Labs outside of LabCorp and Quest:

Currently some practitioners who don't have the ability to draw in their office and send directly to the specialty labs needed for processing, have been able to use ARUP reference labs in Utah for certain Biomarker tests. In these situations, practitioners have to rely on collecting labs or draw stations to collect the blood for their patients. For ex: Scripps labs in Calif. will send a C4a to ARUP who then will send on to National Jewish where it is processed correctly. Because of the current changes made by LabCorp and Quest the information below has been helpful when attention to these details have been strictly followed.

Check MOLD ILLNESS Facebook Page for ongoing updates.

Practitioners need to be acutely aware of the points below when using labs that must send out to one or more facilities for processing:

1. Contracts and or accounts need to be clearly in place between the collection facility and ARUP. It also may be required for the collection facility to have an account or contract with the end processing lab as well for billing purposes. In the above example the end processing lab would be National Jewish. This step if not previously established has been successfully accomplished through the efforts of the Certified Practitioner and the laboratory managers.

2. These tests are unique and have special run codes assigned to them for sending on to another facility from ARUP. These codes must be clarified by the ordering practitioner with the collecting lab and ARUP to be certain that the proper code delivers the specimen to the correct processing facility and that

the collection lab obtains and prepares the specimen correctly to be shipped. This can be readily obtained through the laboratory manager and the Certified Practitioner. Typically, customer service representatives and technicians are not familiar with this information because they are not common tests.

The above two steps must be conducted and verified by the Practitioner and office staff prior to sending patients for draws when utilized.

An example of a biomarker test that can go through ARUP, from a collecting lab to an additional processing facility, would be C4a.

LOW AMYLOSE DIET

FORBIDDEN FOODS:

- Roots and tubers including white and sweet potatoes, beets, peanuts, carrots, and other vegetables which grow under-ground. Onions and garlic are permitted.

- Bananas (the only forbidden fruit).

- Wheat and wheat-based products, including bread, pasta, cakes, crackers, cookies.

- Rice.

- Oats.

- Barley.

- Rye.

- Foods with added sugar, sucrose, corn syrup, or maltodextrin.

ALLOWED FOODS:

Allowed foods include basically anything that is **not** on the list of forbidden foods including:

- Corn.

- Onions.

- Garlic.

- All vegetables that grow above the ground: including lettuce, tomatoes, beans, of all types, peas, cucumbers, and celery.

- All fruits except bananas.

- Meat, fish, and poultry (use "clean" sources)

- Condiments (avoid low-fat varieties as they usually contain added sugar).

- Spices.

- Eggs.

- Dairy (avoid sugar-laden products).

- Nuts.

- Sunflower, pumpkin, and squash seeds.

If you have been advised to be on a gluten-free diet, no changes need to be made in order for you to eat gluten-free. The low amylose diet does **not** allow rice. Gluten-free products often use rice as a substitute for wheat, so read labels carefully.

MEDICAL/
ENVIRONMENTAL TIMELINE

(Start with most recent)

Name: _____ **DOB:** _____

Date: _____ **Health Condition/Diagnosis** _____

Doctor: _____ Tests: _____

Living Environ: _____ Working Environ: _____

Symptoms:

_____

_____

Treatments:

_____

_____

Date: _____ **Health Condition/Diagnosis** _____

Doctor: _____ Tests: _____

Living Environ: _____ Working Environ: _____

Symptoms:

_____

_____

Treatments:

_____

_____

Date: _____ **Health Condition/Diagnosis** _____

Doctor: _____ Tests: _____

Living Environ: _____ Working Environ: _____

Symptoms:

_____

_____

Treatments:

_____

_____

Date: _____ **Health Condition/Diagnosis** _____

Doctor: _____ Tests: _____

Living Environ: _____ Working Environ: _____

Symptoms:

_____

_____

Treatments:

_____

_____

Date: _____ **Health Condition/Diagnosis** _____

Doctor: _____ Tests: _____

Living Environ: _____ Working Environ: _____

Symptoms:

_____

_____

Treatments:

_____

_____

MEDICATION INSTRUCTIONS

COLLOIDAL SILVER/ EDTA/ MUCOLOX NASAL SPRAY

This nasal spray, after much clinical testing and validation, has replaced BEG Spray as the primary treatment of MARCoNS. (BEG is an acronym for Bactroban (mupirocin), EDTA and Gentamicin.) The EDTA dissolves the sticky biofilm produced by the MARCoNS bacteria as a "shield." This allows the concentrated colloidal silver to gain effective access to the bacteria, so they can be eliminated. Mucolox is a polymer that allows the spray to "stick to" the mucous membranes in the sinuses for prolonged contact. This spray is less irritating than the previously used BEG Spray.

Two sprays in each nostril, 3 times a day for 30 days usually is sufficient to eradicate MARCoNS. For children, we generally use 1 spray twice a day. It is **important to be consistent with the dosage**. Skipping a dose here and there will sabotage the effectiveness of the treatment. Remember that CSM should be used for 30 days prior to beginning the compounded Nasal Spray.

EDTA/Colloidal Silver/Mucolox spray does NOT need to be refrigerated.

Your nasal spray comes in a bottle with an actuated nasal sprayer included. The nasal sprayer should be inserted into the bottle intact. Do NOT cut the spray tube.

When using the bottle for the first time (or if you haven't used it for some time) you must prime the pump. Point spray tip away from you then quickly press & release pump. Repeat until a fine spray appears.

In order to get the greatest benefit from your Nasal Spray:

1. Gently blow your nose before spraying so that the spray will penetrate effectively.

2. Remove the cap from the spray tip.

3. Keep the bottle upright.

4. Shake well and gently insert spray tip into nostril. Use the finger of your other hand to close off the other nostril.

5. Bend your head forward.

6. Start to breathe in through your nose while pressing down firmly 1 time on the spray tip.

7. Breathe out through your mouth. Then do the 2nd spray in that nostril.

8. Repeat steps 3 thru 7 for other nostril.

9. Do NOT blow your nose for at least 5 minutes after using the spray.

If the nose becomes irritated, it is suggested that you use vitamin E oil or coconut oil in and around the nostrils between doses of the spray. Apply gently with your little finger or with a cotton swab liberally coated with the oil.

It is essential to re-check the nasal culture 5 to 10 days after the nasal spray treatment is finished, in order to determine if the therapy was effective. Occasionally, a second course of therapy may be required.

EDTA Nasal Spray – Instructions

In some cases, treatment with plain EDTA is sufficient to break down the biofilms that protect bacteria from attack by our own immune system. The course of treatment is usually longer than for the Colloidal Silver Spray

If your practitioner has ordered EDTA Spray for you (usually after a course of EDTA/Silver/Mucolox Spray) **follow the SAME instructions listed above for how to get the most benefit from your Nasal Spray.**

Do not skip doses. It is essential to use the EDTA Spray as directed, for the entire duration of therapy. A MARCoNS culture should be repeated 5 to 10 days after the EDTA treatment is complete.

NEVER assume that MARCoNS is gone, based on symptoms alone.

CHOLESTYRAMINE (CSM)

Cholestyramine (CSM) is an FDA-approved medication originally used to lower elevated levels of cholesterol. It has been used safely for over forty years in millions of patients who have taken the medication for extended periods of time. You have been given a prescription for CSM to be used for only a short period of time to treat your chronic, biotoxin-associated illness.

Cholestyramine is not absorbed from the GI system. Provided that CSM is not taken with food, it binds cholesterol, bile salts and biotoxins in the small intestine. Because it binds biotoxins tightly, the toxins cannot be reabsorbed and are excreted harmlessly in the stool. **CSM has a unique affinity for binding biotoxins. The CSM molecule has a strong positive charge and effectively bonds to the negatively charged biotoxin.** Provided there is no re-exposure to sources of biotoxin, the CSM treatment will remove these toxins from the body over time.

Used at the FDA approved dose, there are gastrointestinal side effects that are potentially annoying but are usually not dangerous and should not interfere with your treatment program. Individuals who tend to be constipated, even before using CSM, will need to be very careful to prevent their stools from becoming too hard. Our treatment protocol attempts to anticipate the possible troublesome side effects; you will be given suggestions for remedies to keep on hand "just in case."

Many patients find that supplementing with high dose fish oil (2400 mg EPA & 1800 mg DHA daily) for 1-2 weeks before starting CSM, as well as during the therapy, will minimize the GI side effects. Fish oils can also help with potential intensification symptoms, sometimes seen with biotoxin mobilization. This phenomenon is especially common in patients with Lyme disease.

Reflux of stomach acid or indigestion is commonly experienced early on in treatment. The symptom resolves spontaneously in most patients within a few days. Mixing the CSM in apple juice, cranberry juice or dissolving CSM, first in lukewarm water and then adding ice, helps reduce heartburn. Bloating and belching can also be caused initially by CSM.

Some individuals will benefit from starting the CSM dosage slowly and building up to the full dose over the course of a few weeks. Many will do well with ½ tsp twice daily to start, increasing by ½ tsp. every 3 to 4 days.

Often, patients simply increase their consumption of fruit or fiber products, such a psyllium (Metamucil), to avoid constipation. Adequate water intake is essential. Magnesium citrate 400 to 800 mg at bedtime can also help to prevent constipation. In stubborn cases, Miralax, an over the counter medication, can hold water in stools, making bowel movements soft and preventing constipation. Because many patients with chronic biotoxin illnesses have diarrhea or frequent soft stools, the constipating side effect of CSM can be a welcome benefit.

CSM has been extensively tested in multiple clinical trials involving patients with chronic, biotoxin illnesses, including CIRS-WDB. **The benefit of using CSM has been confirmed by two double-blind, placebo-controlled crossover studies.**

NOTE: To date there have been no published scientific studies demonstrating benefit from CSM substitutes such as charcoal, chitosan, clay in several forms, or any herbal remedy.

This is likely due to the electrical affinity of CSM for the negatively charged biotoxins found in CIRS-WDB, Post-Lyme, brown recluse spider bites and ciguatera. Think of Velcro. Dense nylon hooks (+) interlock with the nylon pile (-), but two pieces of Velcro with the same surface will not form a bond. CSM is (+) and binds tightly with biotoxins which are (-). Charcoal, chitosan and clay have the same (-) charge as the biotoxins, therefore a strong bond is not likely.

We will use Welchol as a CSM substitute for those unable to take CSM. It is taken with food in a pill form. **It is easier to take but it is only 25% as effective as CSM.**

CSM Protocol:

1. On an empty stomach, take one scoop of CSM (or less if building up to full dose) and mix with 4-6 oz. water or juice.

2. Stir well and swallow. Add more liquid and repeat until all CSM in the glass is consumed. (Do not allow the mixture to sit or it will congeal.)

3. Drink an extra 4-6 oz. of liquid after the CSM.

4. Rinse mouth well or brush teeth after taking CSM. It may stick to the teeth and damage the tooth enamel.

5. After 30 minutes, you may eat or take meds (wait at least 2 hours before taking thyroxine, digitalis, theophylline, Coumadin and others; ask your doctor regarding your specific drugs).

6. Take CSM 4 times a day. (You may start with fewer doses, initially.)

7. If you eat first, wait at least 60 minutes before taking your CSM.

8. Reflux, constipation, bloating and bowel distress are not unusual.

9. Start with lower dose of CSM and increase slowly as needed.

10. Use extra water along with fiber supplements, prunes, magnesium citrate or Miralax, as needed, for constipation.

VIP SPRAY

VIP is a naturally occurring human hormone, which affects multiple pathways in the brain and throughout the body. It improves intracellular energy, reduces pulmonary pressure in exercise, lowers C4a, and stabilizes TGFB-1. It normalizes low VEGF; stabilizes aromatase and helps correct abnormal Vitamin D physiology. **Preliminary genomics testing suggests that VIP may "turn off" the genetic "switch" responsible for CIRS. While further research is needed, VIP has the potential of being a "miracle drug."**

Certified CIRS Practitioners have seen significant improvement in quality of life and stabilization of inflammatory markers in hundreds of patients who have used VIP since November 2008.

In order to use VIP, there are three criteria that each patient must meet:

1. You must Pass the VCS test
2. You must be OUT of Exposure
3. Current MARCoNS test must be Negative.

NOTE: Serum lipase must be checked just prior to VIP and repeated after 30 days of VIP therapy. The initial "test dose" is done in the medical office. TGFB-1 is drawn just before the dose and repeated 30 minutes after the test dose, to rule out current biotoxin exposure.

The VIP spray comes in a light resistant bottle with a metered nasal sprayer included. Each spray delivers 50 mcg of VIP.

The spray bottle is partially filled and contains 12 ml. of VIP, providing 120 sprays. (4 daily doses for 30 days) The usual dose is 1 spray, in a single nostril, 4 times daily (alternate nostrils) **NOTE: Your Certified Practitioner will determine the duration of your VIP Therapy. It will vary depending on your individual response, measured by symptoms, biomarkers, VCS, and genomic testing.**

To get the greatest benefit from your VIP Spray:

VIP must be kept refrigerated and the vial of VIP should be kept upright in the refrigerator to avoid leakage. (Do NOT Freeze.)

VIP must be fresh. Any VIP spray older than one month loses some of its efficacy. Discard unused spray by the expiration date on the label

The nasal sprayer attachment should be inserted into the bottle intact – **Do not cut the tube attached to the sprayer!**

When you first use the bottle (or if you haven't used it for some time), you must **prime the pump**. Point the spray tip away from you and firmly press & release the pump. Repeat until a fine spray appears.

Typically, patients will take their VIP spray when they brush their teeth in the morning and at bedtime as well as at lunch and supper. It does not matter which side of the nose you use and it is not necessary to have the doses spread out exactly 6 hours apart.

1. Gently blow your nose.
2. Remove the cap from the spray tip.
3. Keep the bottle upright.
4. Gently insert the spray tip into nostril. Use the finger of your other hand to close off your other nostril.
5. Bend your head forward.
6. Breathe in through your nose while pressing down firmly 1 time on the spray tip.
7. Breathe out through your mouth.
8. Do NOT blow your nose for 5 minutes after using the VIP spray.

Your Certified Practitioner will need to monitor specific laboratory testing, before and during VIP therapy, to evaluate safety and efficacy.

NOTE: In special circumstances, a diluted solution of VIP may be used on a graduated schedule. Only your Certified CIRS Provider can determine if this option is appropriate for you.

PRIMARY CARE PROVIDERS

OVERVIEW OF THE SHOEMAKER PROTOCOL

The phenomenon of "Mold Illness" has gained increased attention in the past year, but the condition is not new. Dr. Richie Shoemaker, pioneer and visionary in the field of Chronic Inflammatory Response Syndrome (CIRS), has been researching the subject for 18 years. He has identified and documented the etiology, physiological dysregulation, objective clinical manifestations, specific laboratory markers, and effective treatment of this previously elusive syndrome.

The following protocol has evolved from experience with more than 10,000 patients. Compelling scientific data has been meticulously measured, documented and published in peer-reviewed journals, to shed light on a phenomenon that may potentially impact up to 25% of the population.

Patients are encouraged to partner with Shoemaker Certified Practitioners who are experts at diagnosing and treating them systematically, according to this evidence based protocol. With appropriate diagnosis, education, treatment and support, CIRS patients can not only survive, but also THRIVE as they recover their health.

The process requires serious commitment and dedication of both patient and practitioner. The reward, for the vast majority of CIRS patients, is a quality of life that they have not experienced for years, and that many had lost hope of seeing again. The roadmap to success has been validated and will continue to evolve with new scientific discovery and understanding.

The following Protocol is to be followed PRECISELY and SEQUENTIALLY. Each step exists for a specific and scientifically validated reason. Any deviation from the Protocol is likely to impede clinical progress. It is suggested that extraneous supportive interventions be kept to a minimum until the underlying dysregulation

of immune and inflammatory pathways had been corrected and validated by the appropriate biomarkers.

1. Differential Diagnosis is the first step on the road to recovery. Many CIRS patients are misdiagnosed multiple times due to lack of a comprehensive and meticulous history, physical exam, and laboratory assessment. Labels like CFS, fibromyalgia, depression, MS or "somatization" are meaningless without a differential diagnosis that includes CIRS.

A systematic and detailed history is often the key to recognizing CIRS. The standardized Symptom Cluster Analysis is used as a format for interviewing the patient. 37 distinct symptoms, grouped in 13 clusters are carefully explored with the patient. Positive findings in 8 of the 13 clusters suggest the presence of CIRS. This instrument is NOT to be given to the patient for independent completion, as nuances of symptoms may be missed.

A comprehensive medical history includes previous medical diagnoses, medications, supplements, surgeries, major injuries, hospitalizations, and allergies. A developmental and behavioral assessment includes pregnancy complications, school performance, behavioral anomalies and mood volatility.

A thorough environmental history is critical. Any potential (past or present) exposure to Water Damaged Buildings (WDB), molds, herbicides, pesticides, petrochemicals, known toxins or other volatile organic compounds are documented. Any known tick bite or high-risk activities such as hiking, camping, gardening, especially in endemic areas, is noted. History of exposure to toxin-carrying fish or algae blooms is also questioned.

Family medical history and pertinent symptoms are also elicited. It is helpful to have a family member present for this interview. The patient may have limited recall due to cognitive effects of CIRS. The triggering event for CIRS may be recent, or may have occurred years previously. Once triggered, the toxins will remain, in genetically susceptible individuals, until properly treated.

A complete physical exam is conducted to assess for any confounding illness. Specific physical findings common in CIRS include pallor, cool hands or feet, dermatographia, weakness of shoulder anti-gravity muscles with normal grip and shrug strength, malar rash, mild dehydration, postural hypotension, bilateral conjunctival injection and tearing, resting tremor, abnormal gait, and a particular sub-set will be tall and thin with hyper-flexibility.

Visual Contrast Sensitivity (VCS) testing, a scientific tool for evaluating neuro-toxicity caused by biotoxins, is conducted to establish a baseline and repeated after each step of the protocol to monitor clinical progress. Improvement in VCS occurs as the toxin burden is reduced. A regression in VCS is evidence of re-exposure to a biotoxin. Worsening in the VCS scores can be seen within 24 – 36 hours after acute exposure. The VCS may also be impacted by VOC's in susceptible CIRS patients.

An extensive blood profile is drawn to look for HLA-DR and characteristic inflammatory markers that are unique to CIRS. These include HLA-DRB1, DRB3, DRB4, DRB5 and DQB1, C3a, C4a, MSH, MMP-9, TGF beta-1, ADH/Osmolality, VEGF, and VIP. Additional labs, to rule out potential confounding conditions, are also obtained. These generally include anti-gliadin antibodies, anti-cardiolipin antibodies, Cortisol, DHEA, CMP, CBC, CRP, ACTH, TSH, Testosterone, Lipid Profile, Vitamin D3, Leptin, CD4/CD25, and von Willebrand factor. The Progene CIRS Assay, a comprehensive diagnostic test based on proteogenomic analysis, identifies proteins and/or genes that are differentially expressed in subjects suffering from CIRS compared to healthy subjects. It provides a valuable baseline at the time of diagnosis and a unique barometer of clinical success at the end of the Protocol.

If Lyme disease is part of the differential diagnosis, a Western Blot is drawn. Biomarkers including C4a, TGF beta-1, MSH, MMP9, VEGF and VIP are measured repeatedly as the patient progresses through the sequential steps of the Protocol in order to objectively measure and document clinical progress.

NOTE: Some Biomarker labs, especially C4a and TGFB1, are extremely sensitive and must be drawn, processed, shipped and analyzed under precise conditions. Specific labs MUST be utilized for accuracy of results. Do NOT order these labs without verifying the provider with a Certified Practitioner.

A non-contrast MRI with NeuroQuant is utilized to demonstrate predictable brain changes that are caused by the disruption in blood brain barrier that occurs in CIRS. NeuroQuant is a volumetric computer program applied to the brain MRI. Mold exposure is reflected by the unique "fingerprint" of microscopic interstitial edema of white matter in the forebrain and cerebellum, as well as gray matter atrophy and decrease in volume of the caudate nucleus.

Spirometry is performed as part of the initial evaluation. FVC, FEV1, O2 saturation, and FEV1/FVC % are measured. Restrictive lung disease is commonly seen in CIRS. FVC will be reduced and FEV1 to FVC ratio will be normal or elevated in restrictive pulmonary disease. Spirometry is re-evaluated periodically for objective improvement as biomarkers are corrected. A deep nasal culture for multiple antibiotic resistant coagulase negative staph (MARCoNS) is also obtained at the first visit if CIRS is suspected.

---

2. Perform MSQPCR (mold-specific quantitative polymerase chain reaction) fungal DNA testing to ensure there is no ongoing exposure to water damaged buildings. The QPCR is an objective, standardized DNA based method of identifying and quantifying molds. **ERMI (Environmental Relative Moldiness Index) Testing** tests for 36 species and is currently the best predictor of total mold burden. ERMI should be <2 if the patient's C4a less than 20,000. If the C4a is more than 20,000, the ERMI must be a negative 1. The "HERTSMI-2" score looks at 5 organisms from group I in ERMI and assigns weight to the values. Any score over 10 is a problem. NOTE: These numbers are general guidelines. Some patients will remain symptomatic even once these values are obtained. Building performance must be evaluated and optimized as an integral part of this process, in order for patients to obtain and continue clinical success.

3. Remove from exposure to Water Damaged Buildings. Continued exposure to a WDB (home, work, school, etc.) will sabotage patient recovery. This must be stressed to patients and families. Toxins cannot be removed efficiently and physiology corrected if biotoxin exposure is ongoing. Patients who have been dealing with the illness for a longer period, and have been triggered numerous times by WDB, may exhibit a "sicker quicker" phenomenon. Auto activation of MASP-2 results in increased C4a with profound diffuse inflammation and capillary hypo-perfusion. As little as 10 minutes exposure is capable of activating innate immunity & unleashing a predictable cascade of potentially devastating inflammation. Vigilant environmental monitoring and appropriate avoidance is critical to clinical recovery. If the patient is considering moving to a new building, temporarily or permanently, it is essential to do a QPCR evaluation on the new structure prior to relocating. Proper decontamination of contents is critical. Porous items such as mattresses, upholstered furniture, and paper items will invariably need to be replaced. Clothing may be machine washed or dry cleaned using appropriate precautions.

4. Reduce biotoxin load in the body with Cholestryamine 4 grams on an empty stomach 4 times daily. Medically frail or sensitive individuals will likely need to start with smaller amounts and ramp up gradually to a full dose. (Some patients will only be able to tolerate 1/4 tsp. daily to start.) In very sensitive individuals, CSM may be preceded by 1 week of high-dose fish oils and a low amylose diet. (See Appendix). This therapy is continued for at least 5 days after CSM is started. These interventions are to reduce the chances of an intensification reaction from CSM. Patients are given an instruction sheet on proper use and timing of CSM in relation to medications, supplements and food (See Appendix).

Use Welchol 2 tablets three times daily, with food, for those who do not tolerate CSM. Welchol is only ¼ as effective in binding capacity. Compliance may be facilitated by using CSM in the morning and at bedtime and Welchol with lunch and dinner. Monitor progress with VCS vision test. Once the patient has passed the VCS test, or taken the CSM for 1 month, the next step of the protocol, treatment of MARCoNS, can begin.

NOTE: At the end of the protocol, patients are instructed in the prophylactic use of CSM or Welchol for potential re-exposure.

---

5. Eradicate biofilm forming Multiply Antibiotic Resistant Coagulase Negative Staphylococcus (MARCoNS), detected by deep nasal culture. (See manual for nasal culture procedure). If the API-Staph culture (specific for coagulase negative staph) shows resistance to two or more distinct classes of antibiotics, give EDTA/Colloidal Silver/Mucolox Spray ,2 sprays in each nostril tid for 1 month. A repeat culture is taken 1 week after completing BEG spray. Persistent MARCoNS is treated with plain EDTA, 2 sprays in each nostril three times daily for 6-8 weeks, to dissolve stubborn biofilms. Re-culture is performed after 1 week off the spray. If MARCoNS persists after the above steps, consider canine exposure, close contact with another person with low MSH or ongoing environmental exposure. MARCoNS exists in the presence of a low MSH. Once MSH is levels are corrected, the opportunistic organisms should not return unless there is re-exposure and relapse.

6. Correct anti-gliadin antibodies (AGA) by avoiding gluten-containing foods for at least 3 months. Low MSH causes dysregulation of T-reg cells with the potential development of autoimmune disorders. Re-check AGA after 3 months and, if negative, the patient may cautiously and gradually re-introduce gluten into the diet, while documenting re-emergence of any symptoms. If AGA is still positive, celiac disease must be ruled out. If Tissue Transglutaminase (TTG) antibodies are elevated, gluten is permanently eliminated. NOTE: Many patients will feel better without gluten, even when the TTG antibodies are normal.

7. Correct androgens. Abnormal androgens are commonly caused by up-regulation of aromatase. If DHEA is low, supplement DHEA, up to 25 mg. three times daily for one month. Estradiol levels are checked after two weeks on DHEA. Excess aromatase activity will be corrected by VIP later in the protocol. Treatment with testosterone is contraindicated, at this stage, as up-regulated aromatase activity will promote conversion of testosterone to estrogen.

8. Correct elevated MMP9. Matrix Metalloproteinase 9 is an enzyme that disrupts the basement membrane of endothelial cells, increasing vascular permeability and allowing inflammatory compounds to enter the brain, nerves, muscles, joints and lungs. This enzyme significantly weakens the blood brain barrier and may cause debilitating neurological symptoms, seen in the most compromised CIRS patients. If MMP9 is elevated (over 332ng/ml) it is treated with a low amylose diet and high dose fish oil (2.4 gm. EPA and 1.8 gm. DHA total daily dose).

9. Correct ADH / Osmolality. Biotoxin patients often experience a low ADH and an increased serum osmolality due to the inability of the kidneys to hold on to free water. Symptoms include polydipsia, polyuria, postural hypotension, migraine-like headaches, and frequent static shocks. Low ADH/high osmolality may mimic Postural Orthostatic Tachycardia Syndrome (POTS). These symptoms may include fatigue, headaches, lightheadedness, heart palpitations, exercise intolerance, nausea, diminished concentration, tremors, syncope cold extremities, chest pain and dyspnea. Low ADH is treated with desmopressin (DDAVP) 0.2 mg every other day, at bedtime, for 2 weeks. Serum sodium is checked in 5 days and again at 10 days to monitor for hyponatremia. Daily weights and weekly electrolyte monitoring is indicated if DDAVP therapy is potentially required longer than 2 weeks.

10. Correct VEGF. Vascular Endothelial Growth Factor stimulates angiogenesis in response to Hypoxia Inducible Factor and promotes capillary vasodilatation. VEGF is often suppressed (less than 31 pg/ml) in patients with CIRS. This results in capillary hypo-perfusion and diffuse tissue hypoxia. Symptoms of "brain fog", fatigue, muscle pain, dyspnea on exertion and post-exercise exhaustion are often associated with a low VEGF. It is treated with a low amylose diet and high dose fish oil (see Step 8 above).

11. Correct elevated Complement C3a. This split product of complement activation is elevated in the presence of bacterial membranes, such as Borrelia. If elevated, the bacterial infection is first treated with antibiotics. If C3a remains elevated, after all prior interventions, a statin can be used to lower the level. Zocor 80 mg/day is given for a limited period, along with CoQ10 150 mg/day. 10 days of CoQ10 therapy, prior to starting Zocor, is suggested to minimize side effects due to reduced levels of ubiquinone. Liver enzymes are evaluated prior to starting statins and repeated in 1 month.

12. Correct elevated Complement C4a if levels are greater than 2830 ng/ml. C4a is also a split product of complement activation and a potent anaphylatoxin. Elevation is due to the diffuse inflammation caused by CIRS-WDB. C4a is a critical marker that indicates the acute severity of the syndrome. VIP (Vasoactive Intestinal Polypeptide) is the treatment of choice. It is a nasal spray, dosed at 50 mcg/ml, 1 spray 4 times daily. (See Step #14 for guidelines.) Older treatment regimens that employed mini-dose erythropoietin are no longer recommended.

13. Correct elevated TGFB-1. Transforming Growth Factor Beta-1 causes dysfunctional tissue remodeling. It down-regulates VEGF and influences T-reg cells to induce autoimmunity. A CIRS specific T-Reg Cell Panel (CD4+CD25++CD127 lo/-) may be ordered to evaluate pathologic immune response. If TGF-B1 remains elevated (over 2380 pg/ml) after the previous steps of the protocol have been implemented, you may treat with losartan, beginning at 12.5 to 25 mg daily. (This therapy is not used if the patient is hypotensive.) Once blood pressure is stabilized, increase to 25 mg bid for 30 days. A metabolite, specific to losartan, (exp 3179), lowers TGF-B1 levels. Blood pressure monitoring is important during therapy, especially for patients already on anti-hypertensive agents.

14. Correct low Vasoactive Intestinal Polypeptide (VIP) if the patient is still symptomatic after the above steps. The fundamental goal of CIRS Treatment is to restore the regulation of the innate immune system. Some patients will achieve this goal before completing all the sequential steps of the Protocol. For those who are still symptomatic at this stage, VIP offers real hope. The nasal spray is dosed at 50 mcg/ml, 1 spray 4 times daily. The first dose is given in the office. A TGF-B1 level is drawn prior to the VIP administration and again 15 minutes later. If there is a rise in TGF-B1, it is an indication of hidden mold exposure. It is critical that there be no continued mold exposure, that MARCoNS culture be negative and VCS testing is normal before starting VIP. When those conditions are met, VIP has the ability to correct C4a, TGF-B1, VEGF, MMP9, estradiol, testosterone, Vitamin D3 and Pulmonary Artery Systolic Pressure. It can dramatically improve quality of life. Serum lipase is tested prior to beginning VIP, and monthly during VIP therapy. If there is a significant rise in lipase, determine the cause as this may require the cessation of VIP therapy.

15. Monitor stability of clinical symptoms & laboratory tests off of medications. Vigilance concerning re-exposure is essential. Patients are instructed in prophylactic use of CSM or Welchol for potential re-exposure.

Dr. Shoemaker's depiction of the Biotoxin Pathway has given us a previously unappreciated view of innate immunity and the cascade of dysregulation caused by biotoxins and related inflammagens in genetically susceptible individuals. Ongoing research on the genomics of CIRS, by Dr. Shoemaker and Dr. Ryan, continues to expand our understanding of this very prevalent syndrome and its successful clinical management.

Having a Primary Care Provider (PCP) who is informed about the Shoemaker Protocol is extremely valuable. While the initial diagnosis and active management of CIRS should be done by a Certified CIRS Practitioner, the PCP will be able to provide essential follow-up and integration of care.

A PCP who does not understand the multi-system, multi-symptom picture of CIRS, often treats the mosaic of seemingly unrelated symptoms with therapies that are fundamentally unsuccessful, in the long term. Once the Shoemaker Protocol is followed precisely, the inflammatory cascade halted, and biomarkers normalized, symptoms are generally resolved. Those that remain may be due to a co-existing issue.

RE-EXPOSURE CHALLENGES CRITICAL OBSERVATION SKILLS

"MOLDY"

Below are basic observational skills for deciding whether to enter a building based on the acronym MOLDY:

M- Musty smell - If you smell musty smells when you walk in, leave **IMMEDIATELY**!

O- Old Buildings- The best chance of being safe is with buildings between 2 and 12 years old. Nearly all buildings 20+ yrs. old will have had some water intrusion event.

L- Look for Leaking- water stained or missing ceiling tiles, rippled or buckling floors, wrinkling wallpaper. New paint on part of a wall or ceiling could be hiding a water stain from a leak. Moisture on the inside of a window or door with or without watermarks can be a danger sign.

D- Discoloration- look for discoloration and stains on surfaces, such as wood cabinets, wood ceilings, grout or tile in a bathroom, walls, floors, and ceilings.

Y- Yield to these observations and become diligent in recognizing them! The harsh reality is that if this kind of tangible evidence is observed in a building, a CIRS patient should not go inside. Grocery stores, restaurants, movie theaters, offices, and other commercial buildings must be assumed to be moldy until proven otherwise.

If you choose to enter a building you have not been in before, that passes the basic observation skills listed here, it is important to carefully monitor your symptoms for the next few minutes, then over the next 24 to 72 hours. There are buildings that may not have obvious signs of water damage but can still expose you to mold toxins and other inflammatory chemicals that produce delayed symptoms. Repeated exposure to "less sick" buildings can still be harmful over time. These buildings pose the greatest challenge because of the less obvious signs, and the delay in onset of symptoms.

QUESTIONS TO ASK WHEN TRAVELING

T- Talk – Ask to talk with a knowledgeable manger, maintenance person, or someone who knows the history of the building in which you would like to stay or visit.

R- Reaction/Response- When talking to a person with the most knowledge about the building, let them know that **you have a strong and potentially immediate immune reaction/response to any building that has had a water intrusion event or any kind of water damage**. Examples include problems with plumbing, roof leaks, and fire sprinkler malfunctions, to name a few. **Never ask, "Have you had any problems with mold?" This, unfortunately, puts people on the defensive**.

A- Avoid- Let the person you are talking with know you must avoid staying in a building that has had any issues with water damage. Without being critical or demanding, be assertive enough to get the facts you need without judgment. Avoid any hotel or building that has indoor water features such as fountains, waterfalls, or open terrariums.

V- Validate any Visible signs witnessed or prior events of water damage that you are being told about. When asked if any water intrusion has occurred, the manager responded with, "Not really, we just had a small leak from a plumbing issue with a bathtub that went between the 2nd and 1st floors. It's all been taken care of." Many people assume unless the water event was a major flood that these kinds of things don't matter, but they really **DO** for the CIRS patient!

E- Equip yourself with the Evidence you need to make a logical and informed choice about the building you are inquiring about.

L-Let go. If there is no one that is willing or able to talk with you about the history of the building or if any water damage has occurred, it is best to let go and move on to another alternative.

"SCRIPTS" FOR COMMUNICATING YOUR SPECIFIC NEEDS

There are a number of predictable scenarios that will occur as you navigate through daily life with CIRS. Anticipating these challenges, and being prepared for them, is the key to preventing unnecessary exposure. If a particular building is not safe for you, but you require the services of the business, a simple "script" can help you to communicate outside the building.

A brief encounter with someone does not have to go into every detail. Describing enough of the situation, in a way that encourages a helpful response, is all that is needed. This can often become an opportunity to educate those who want to learn more.

Following are the proactive "scripts" you can adapt to your unique situation.

Script 1: Brief Explanation of CIRS:

The subject of CIRS may come up in a **social situation where you only have a minute or two describe your illness**. This brief statement helps you to get the main points across.

"My immune system is not working properly. I have an extreme response to mold toxins that come from water damaged buildings. I inherited a gene that keeps my immune system on constant 'alert' when exposed to these toxins. My body is not able to eliminate them like most people can. I have to be extremely careful to not enter buildings that have had water damage.

My own immune system causes severe inflammation throughout my body in response to these toxins. This causes severe fatigue, brain fog, muscle pain, shortness of breath, and other physical symptoms for me. I am in treatment, but it is not a quick fix."

Script 2: Conversation with Retail Employee:

(You have entered a newer building that passed the "MOLDY" criteria)

"Hello, May I ask you a question?"

"Sure"

"Do you know if this building has had any kind of water intrusion or water damage?"

"Yes, we have had some roof leaks from the storms we had this winter. I think they are all fixed now."

"Thank you. I have a medical condition where I have a severe immune response to a building that has had any kind of water damage. I'm not able to stay inside the building. I do need to purchase something. Would you be able to help me outside?"

"Yes, we can have someone bring that product out for you and collect payment there."

"Thank you, I really appreciate it!"

When this employee came outside to help me, she inquired more about what caused me to have a physical problem when a building had been water damaged. I was able to briefly provide information about CIRS and the website for her to go to. This person has a relative who had been chronically ill and was known to live in a house that had visible mold.

End Result: Crisis averted and valuable information given that might help the employee's family!

Note: If the building had NOT had a history of water damage, you would be able to remain inside to conduct your business and then TRACK your exposure to that building on your Tracking Form, in the event of a delayed reaction to unknown biotoxins.

SAMPLE LETTERS RE: CIRS

EMPLOYER

To Whom It May Concern:

_____ is a patient of mine. He/She has been diagnosed with Chronic Inflammatory Response Syndrome (CIRS) as a result of exposure to water damaged buildings. He/She has a particular genetic susceptibility to this condition and multiple specific lab findings that confirm his/her diagnosis.

_____ is in active treatment and it is imperative that he/she work in a safe environment that has been verified by testing for DNA evidence of mold, mold by-products, specific bacterial species, and VOC's. The CIRS standard for this testing is the ERMI test by Mycometrics.

_____ was advised, after careful evaluation of symptom and location tracking sheets, that the work environment is clearly causing an increase in clinical symptoms.

(Specific location) was tested with an ERMI test, according to the medical standard for CIRS patients. The objective analysis of that location was _____.

_____ symptoms are clearly worse when exposed to this area. It is imperative that he/she avoid this area as well as any other areas of the building(s) that may have had any previous water leak, water intrusion, or persistent moisture accumulation. Because the biotoxins are microscopic, and carried by air currents, they may spread widely beyond the original source.

It is imperative that _____ avoid exposure to the contaminates identified by DNA testing. Without this precaution, his/her medical recovery will be in serious jeopardy.

Sincerely,

_____

LANDLORD/HOME SELLER

To Whom It May Concern:

_____is a patient of mine. He/She has been diagnosed with Chronic Inflammatory Response Syndrome (CIRS) as a result of exposure to water damaged buildings. He/She has a particular genetic susceptibility to this condition and multiple laboratory tests which have confirmed this medical diagnosis.

_____ is in active treatment and it is imperative that he/she live in a safe environment that has been tested for DNA evidence of mold as well as mold by-products, specific bacterial species, and VOC's.

I have advised _____to have any potential living environment tested with an ERMI test, according to the medical standard for CIRS patients. Without this precaution, his/her medical recovery will be in serious jeopardy.

Sincerely,

_____

SCHOOL

To Whom It May Concern:

_____ is a patient of mine. He/She has been diagnosed with Chronic Inflammatory Response Syndrome (CIRS) as a result of exposure to water damaged buildings. He/She has a particular genetic susceptibility to this condition and multiple specific lab findings that confirm this diagnosis.

_____ is in currently in active treatment. It is imperative that he/she must be in a safe environment that has been verified by testing for DNA evidence of mold, mold by-products, specific bacterial species, and VOC's. The CIRS standard for this testing is the ERMI test by Mycometrics.

_____ was advised, after careful evaluation of symptom and location tracking sheets, that the school environment is clearly causing an increase in clinical symptoms.

(Specific location) was tested with an ERMI test, according to the medical standard for CIRS patients. The objective analysis of that location was _____.

_____ symptoms are clearly worse when exposed to this area. It is imperative that he/she avoid this area as well as any other areas of the building(s) that may have had any previous water leak, water intrusion, or persistent moisture accumulation. Because the biotoxins are microscopic, and carried by air currents, they may spread widely beyond the original source.

It is imperative that _____ avoid exposure to the contaminates identified by DNA testing. Without this precaution, his/her medical recovery will be in serious jeopardy.

Sincerely,

_____

DAILY TRACKING FORM

INTRODUCTION

Your Immune System can react to: Biotoxins, Chemicals, Bacterial or Viral Exposure, Detoxification Supplements, Immune Stimulants, Anti-biotic, Anti-viral, or Anti-fungal meds or supplements.

The emphasis in tracking is to record CHANGES in activities and CHANGES in symptoms. This will allow you to document cause and effect and determine where your symptoms are coming from. Use the KEY at the bottom of this page.

SYMPTOMS:

Circle the 6 most common or problematic symptoms you are currently experiencing. Then write these in the SYMPTOM column on your Tracking Form. The additional spaces under SYMPTOMS are to list new symptoms that emerge as a result of the CHANGES you make in various activities.

- Aches, am stiffness, fatigue, ice pick pain, joint pain, muscle cramps, tremors, unusual pain, weakness
- Blurred vision, headache, light sensitivity, red eyes, sinus problems, tearing, vertigo
- Cough, shortness of breath
- Abdominal pain, appetite swings, diarrhea, excessive thirst, increased urination, metallic taste,
- Numbness, poor temperature regulation, skin sensitivity (crawling sensation), static shocks, sweats (especially night sweats), tingling,

- Confusion, difficulty learning, disorientation, memory problems, mood swings, poor focus/concentration, word recall issues

LOCATIONS:

ALWAYS assess a building for safety prior to entering, using the MOLDY criteria in the Appendix. List the 5-6 buildings you visit on a regular basis under the LOCATION section. The additional spaces will be used to list buildings you enter on occasion, as this is a CHANGE in your daily routine.

SUPPLEMENTS/MEDS:

Supplements and meds are to be used discriminately. List your current meds and supplements (including dosage)

TREATMENTS/THERAPIES:

If you are doing additional therapies such as massage, acupuncture, detox baths, saunas, or other holistic therapies, list those and note any CHANGES that occur in that routine.

COMMENTS:

_____

_____

_____

_____

KEY

- **Occurrence X**
- **Increase +**
- **Marked Increase ++**
- **Med, Supplement Treatment Started S**
- **Med, Supplement or Treatment Stopped O**
- **Increase in Med or Supplement Dose ^ #**
- IE: Increased from one cap to two caps = ^ 2
- **Decrease in Med or Supplement Dose v #**
- IE: Decreased from two caps to one caps = v 1
- **Event E (exposure to illness, unusual stress, exposure to toxins not related to specific building) Note specific event under "comments."**

The most important reason to track is to record CHANGES in your activities so that you will be able to recognize where your symptoms are coming from.

NOTE: Make copies of the blank tracking form to fill out each week.

EXAMPLE OF COMPLETED TRACKING FORM

DATE: 7-3-17 TO 7-9-17	M	T	W	Th	F	S	S
SPECIFIC LOCATIONS: Where I have been							
1 Home (safe)	X	X	X	X	X	X	X
2 Grocery Store - Martin's Food Outlet (safe)	X						
3 School (Unknown)			X				
4 Church (Unknown)							X
5 Post Office (new)		X					
6 Cleaned boxes in garage (new)			X				
7 Company visited- sick with colds				E			
8							
9							
10							

DATE: 7-3-17 TO 7-9-17	M	T	W	Th	F	S	S
SYMPTOMS:							
1 Brain Fog		X					
2 Muscle Aches	X	X	X+	X++	X+	X	X
3 Joint Pain	X	X	X	X++	X+	X	X
4 Muscle Twitching			X		X+		
5 Fatigue	X	X	X+	X++	X+	X	X
6 Headache				X			
7 Sinus Pressure/Pain (new)				X	X+		
8							
9							
10							

DATE: 7-3-17 TO 7-9-17	M	T	W	Th	F	S	S
SUPPLEMENTS / MEDS: (evaluate regularly for current need)							
1 Probiotic one/day							
2 Omega-3 one 3x/day							
3 Turmeric two caps daily							
4 CSM when needed scoop					S 1	^2	
5 Glutathione spray (new) 2sprays/day			S		O		
6 Liver support formula (new) 2 caps/day			S	O			
7 b-12 drops one cap daily			^2	v 1			
8							
9							
10							

DATE: 7-3-17 TO 7-9-17	M	T	W	Th	F	S	S
TREATMENTS / THERAPIES:							
1 massage twice/month							
2							
3							
4							
5							
6							

Tracking Form

DATE:			M	T	W	Th	F	S	S
SPECIFIC LOCATIONS: Where I have been									
1									
2									
3									
4									
5									
6									
7									
8									
9									
10									

DATE:			M	T	W	Th	F	S	S
SYMPTOMS:									
1									
2									
3									
4									
5									
6									
7									
8									
9									
10									

DATE:			M	T	W	Th	F	S	S
SUPPLEMENTS / MEDS: (evaluate regularly for current need)									
1									
2									
3									
4									
5									
6									
7									
8									
9									
10									

DATE:			M	T	W	Th	F	S	S
TREATMENTS / THERAPIES:									
1									
2									
3									
4									
5									
6									

GLOSSARY

ACQUIRED IMMUNE SYSTEM - Acquired (adaptive) immunity is not present at birth. It is learned as the immune system encounters foreign substances (antigens). Acquired immunity attacks each antigen with a specific antibody and develops a memory for that antigen.

AIR SCRUB- Term used to describe when cleaning the air using a HEPA filtration system

AMYLOSE – a complex plant starch contained primarily in wheat rye, oats, barley, rice, bananas and root vegetables. (SEE Low Amylose Diet in Appendix)

ANDROGENS – male hormones (often dysregulated due to low MSH in individuals with CIRS)

ANTIDIURETIC HORMONE (ADH) - also known as vasopressin, this hormone is made by the posterior pituitary and is responsible for retaining free water from the kidneys. ADH is often reduced with low MSH and should be measured along with serum osmolality for an accurate picture of fluid balance.

ATP- Adenosine Triphosphate is known as the "energy of life" as it exists in all living things. By using ATP meters, one can test the cleanliness of a surface.

BEG SPRAY- a prescription nasal spray consisting of Bactroban, EDTA and Gentamycin used to eradicate MARCoNS . This has been **replaced** by a more effective formula consisting of EDTA, Colloidal Silver and Mucolox.

BIOFILM – a dense biopolymer "slime" produced by a microorganism, such as a bacteria. This "slime" forms a shield that protects the bacteria from attack by the immune system or by antibiotics.

BIOMARKER- a specific lab test that reflects the biological activity of an illness, like CIRS. Some biomarkers will change with effective therapy.

BIOTOXIN- a toxic substance produced by a living organism

BIOTOXIN PATHWAY- the complex dynamic interaction of specific microbes with genetics, cytokines, hormones, and immune factors, which results in CIRS (see diagram of Biotoxin Pathway)

BUILDING PERFORMANCE- Building performance or home performance is a comprehensive whole-house approach to identifying and fixing comfort, indoor air quality, and energy efficiency problems in the built environment.

BUILDING SCIENCE- the collection of scientific knowledge and experience that focuses on the analysis and control of the physical phenomena affecting buildings and architecture.

C3A- Immune system complement protein often elevated in acute Lyme Disease)

C4A- An immune system complement protein and inflammatory marker of great significance in CIRS. C4a reflects innate immune responses in those with exposure to Water Damaged Buildings (WDB). These short-lived proteins are manufactured rapidly, and a rise in blood levels is seen within12 hours of exposure to biotoxins. The elevation will persist until definitive therapy is initiated.

CHOLESTYRAMINE (CSM)- A non-absorbable anion binding resin used to bind biotoxins so that they can be eliminated through the stool.

NOTE: the positive charge of CSM makes it especially effective in binding the negatively charged biotoxins. Charcoal, bentonite clay and other common "binders" are negatively charged, so they do NOT have this property.

CIGUATERA- a toxin-producing dinoflagellate acquired by eating tainted tropical reef dwelling predatory fish

CIRS – WDB – Chronic Inflammatory Response Syndrome caused by exposure to Water Damaged Buildings

COMBUSTION APPLIANCE ZONE- CAZ testing is a health and safety diagnostic that is recommended where combustion appliances are in use.

CRITICAL BARRIERS- dividers usually made from 6-10 mil plastic sheeting to isolate specific areas

CYTOKINES- critical proteins that direct the response of the innate immune system. Dysregulated cytokines cause massive inflammation.

DEPRESSURIZATION- to reduce the air pressures in a given space

DUCT REGISTERS- HVAC system outlet grills that supply air via the duct system.

EDTA/Silver 0.5% /25ppm with 15% Mucolox Nasal Spray – used to eliminate MARCoNS in the presence of a positive nasal culture.

END POINT CRITERIA- Post remediation criteria used to determine a pass or fail, based on the sample results using specified requirements

ERMI- Environmental Relative Moldiness Index is a test requiring analysis of a single sample of dust from a home. The sample is analyzed using a highly specific DNA-based method for quantifying mold species. A simple algorithm is used to calculate a ratio of water damage-related species to common indoor molds and the resulting score is called the ERMI.

EXOTOXINS- a toxin released by a living cell into its surroundings Exotoxins can cause damage to the host by destroying cells or disrupting normal cellular metabolism, including suppressing MSH.

GENETIC SUSCEPTIBILITY- a specific group of immune response genes represented by the HLA-DR on chromosome 6

GENOMICS- the study of the function and interaction of genes and their dynamic relationship with the environment

GLIADIN – a protein contained in gluten

GLUTEN- a protein found primarily in wheat, rye and barley

HEPA- High Efficiency Particulate Air Filter, designed to remove 99.97% of airborne particles measuring 0.3 micrometers or greater in diameter passing through it

HEPA VACUUM- Vacuum cleaner equipped with special filters that capture 99.7% of particles larger than 0.3 microns

HERTSMI-2- HERTSMI-2 is an acronym for Health Effects Roster of Type Specific Formers of Mycotoxins and Inflammagens - 2nd Version. HERTSMI-2 differs from ERMI Testing in its limited focus. HERTSMI-2 Testing looks at 5 mold species while ERMI looks at 36 mold species.

HLA – We inherit a copy of the **Human Leukocyte Antigen** (HLA) -from each biological parent. The immune HLAs are located on chromosome 6 and are predictive of which individuals are genetically susceptible to develop CIRS. (See HLA chart in Appendix)

HOME PERFORMANCE CONTRACTING- licensed, and certified company that contracts to perform a comprehensive whole-house approach identifying and fixing comfort, indoor air quality, and energy efficiency problems in the built environment

INFLAMMAGEN- an irritant that causes a local or generalized response to cellular injury that is marked by capillary dilatation, infiltration of white blood cells, redness, heat, pain, swelling, and often, loss of function

IR CAMERA- a non-contact device that detects infrared energy (heat) and converts it into an electronic signal, which is then processed to produce a thermal image on a video monitor and perform temperature calculations

INNATE IMMUNE SYSTEM – Innate (natural) immunity is present at birth and does not have to be learned through exposure to an invader. It provides an immediate response to foreign invaders as the fundamental "first responder" of the immune system.

INNERWALL CAVITY TESTING- bio-aerosol test that is used to sample the inside of a wall cavity for contaminates

LEAKY GUT- a hyper-permeable intestine. The intestinal lining becomes more porous, with more holes developing that are larger in size. This permits larger, undigested food molecules and other "bad stuff" to flow freely into your bloodstream.

LEPTIN- a cytokine hormone manufactured by fat cells. Leptin activates the production of MSH. High leptin and low MSH are the hallmarks of obesity caused by toxins.

LYME DISEASE- a biotoxin illness caused by the spirochete, Borrelia burgdorferi, carried by ticks

MARCONS- multiply antibiotic resistant coagulase negative staph. These bacteria may colonize the upper nasal passages, especially when MSH is low. MARCoNS stimulate cytokines & exotoxins and contribute to the inflammatory response.

MICROVAC TESTING- bio-aerosol test that is used to sample various porous objects such as carpeting, fabric furnishings, fabric drapes, pillows etc.

MMP9- matrix metalloproteinase #9 is an enzyme that disrupts tissue under the walls of blood vessels. This substance delivers inflammatory chemicals to the brain, nerves, lung, muscles and joints.

MOLD- fungi capable of digesting organic matter. Molds produce and release microscopic spores and mycotoxins which can dramatically impact health, especially in genetically susceptible individuals.

MSH - ALPHA MELANOCYTE STIMULATING HORMONE- Made in the hypothalamus, this hormone controls nerves, hormones, cytokines, and mucus membrane immune defense. MSH also regulates melatonin and endorphin levels affecting restorative sleep, fatigue, pain and mood.

MYCOTOXIN- a biologic toxin made by molds or fungi

NAM- Negative Air Machine used to create negative air pressure

NEGATIVE PRESSURE- An area of lower air pressure, used to isolate an area to prevent cross contamination. This directs air flow to trap unwanted particles.

NEURO-QUANT (NQ)- a computer program, applied to a completed non-contrast brain MRI, which measures the volume of specific brain structures. Changes in sizes of these structures is statistically significant in the diagnosis of CIRS, Traumatic Brain Injury, Lyme Disease, Alzheimer's, and perhaps other brain abnormalities.

OSMOLALITY- the measure of the relative amount of salt and water in the blood or in the urine. Osmolality is a reflection of the degree of hydration.

POST-LYME SYNDROME- persistent symptoms and physiologic abnormalities after adequate antibiotic treatment in patients with a valid Lyme Disease diagnosis. Most often seen in patients with HLA 15-6-51 or 16-5-51 or in patients with multi-susceptibility. Evaluation for CIRS-WDB is indicated.

POSITIVE PRESSURE- Positive pressure is a pressure within a system that is greater than the environment that surrounds that system.

PPE- Personal Protective Equipment including respirator with the appropriate filtration, full suit with hood and booties, gloves, and eye protection.

REMEDIATION- the process of safely removing mold contamination and associated inflammagens from inhabited spaces. **NOTE**: The standards for mold remediation for an individual with CIRS far exceed that of the general population. The detailed work plan should be directed by a CIRS literate environmental professional.

RETURN REGISTER- HVAC system inlet grille(s) that pull air from the building to the furnace or air handler to be heated or cooled then released back into the building via the "supply" ducted registers.

RESERVOIR- potential source for contamination such as carpeting or upholstery

S DOOR- Used to control air pressure in remediation work areas or decontamination areas.

SICK BUILDING SYNDROME- common general term used to describe the illness caused exposure to the toxic environment of a structure with water damage or other chemical toxins or VOC's

TAPE LIFT- method of using a clear tape or slide as a collection medium for sampling contaminates. The sample is analyzed using a microscope.

TGFB-1- **Transforming Growth Factor-** This protein helps control the growth, division, appearance and function of cells. TGF Beta-1 typically elevates dramatically with mold exposure and decreases with removal of toxins. It has the ability to regulate inflammation in multiple body systems. TGFB-1 is a vital biomarker to monitor throughout the recovery process.

TOXIN BURDEN- the accumulation of toxins within the body due to the CIRS patient's genetically determined inability to identify and remove these toxins.

TUMOR NECROSIS FACTOR (TNF)- a cell signaling protein. The primary role of TNF is in the regulation of immune cells.

ULTRASONIC BATH- Ultrasonic Cleaning process that uses ultrasound (usually from 20–400 kHz) and an appropriate cleaning solvent (sometimes ordinary tap water) to clean items. The ultrasound can be used with just water, but use of a solvent appropriate for the item to be cleaned and the type of soiling present enhances the effect.

VCS TEST – VISUAL CONTRAST SENSITIVITY- a specific vision contrast test that measures the neurotoxic deficits in vision seen in patients with CIRS. These deficits reverse as toxins are cleared from the body.

VEGF- Vascular Endothelial Growth Factor promotes growth of new blood vessels to enhance circulation. Low VEGF is common in patients with CIRS, but there may be a compensatory mild elevation of VEGF early in the disease.

VIP – Vasoactive Intestinal Peptide - a neuro-regulatory hormone that regulates cytokine responses, pulmonary artery pressures, and inflammation throughout the body. Low VIP levels are present in CIRS patients and also in patients with multiple chemical sensitivity. This leads to unusual shortness of breath, especially in exercise. In the GI system, low VIP may cause watery diarrhea. VIP plays a role similar to MSH in regulating inflammatory responses. Current research suggests that VIP plays an important in the genomics of CIRS.

VOC'S- Volatile Organic Compounds are organic compounds that easily become vapors or gases. Breathing these substances may have immediate or long-term health consequences for susceptible individuals

WDB- Water Damaged Building.

NOTE: There does not need to be visible mold or obvious water damage. If water intrusion occurred and persisted for at least 48 hours, the conditions exist for a potentially unacceptable & hazardous indoor environment for an individual with CIRS. **WELCHOL-** a medication occasionally used as a binding agent to reduce biotoxins in patients with CIRS (25% as effective as CSM).

ABOUT THE AUTHORS

This Recovery Manual is the result of the efforts of a unique and specialized team of CIRS experts. Their legacy is this important tool, capable of empowering thousands of individuals with CIRS to navigate the road to recovery.

Paula Vetter is a Holistic Family Nurse Practitioner with more than 30 years of experience in both Traditional and Functional Medicine. She was a Critical Care Instructor at the prestigious Cleveland Clinic for more than a decade, taught at two Ohio colleges, and did primary care in a busy Family Practice in NE Ohio. Paula is a Shoemaker Certified CIRS Practitioner who had a private CIRS practice in central CA, until she recently retired. Her passion is educating, inspiring and empowering individuals and families to take charge of their health and transform their lives. Paula, Laurie, and Cindy functioned, in practice, as a cohesive multi-disciplinary team, to successfully treat all aspects of CIRS.

Laurie Rossi is a Registered Nurse with 34 years of practical, "hands on", experience that includes specialties in Oncology, Integrative Medicine, and Patient Education. Laurie is a CIRS patient herself and lives the daily challenges that come with that diagnosis. She has worked personally with Dr. Shoemaker to achieve her own recovery, using his Protocol. Since 2010, she has worked tirelessly to provide information and understanding about CIRS to professionals and patients. She has worked with hundreds of clients with CIRS, in practice and as a patient care advocate, to help them navigate their personal road back to health. Her hope and dream has been to unite a team of compassionate and dedicated professionals to address each of the specific areas of need for the CIRS patient. She feels that God answered her prayer, which culminated in the completion of this manual. Her heart for helping others, along with her unique understanding of living with CIRS, is a tremendous blessing.

Cindy Edwards is a general building contractor, and certified building analyst that specializes in home performance contracting. Cindy has been an amazing colleague who learned about CIRS and the unique standard of practice it takes to be successful with these clients. Cindy saw many clients with CIRS fail, after spending thousands of dollars with "mold experts". She studied extensively and obtained the specialized knowledge necessary to assess buildings, and remediate them successfully. Cindy knew there had to be a better way, so she created it! Now she teaches those skills to others.

This book is the culmination of the heartfelt desire of the authors, to help patients and families as they deal with CIRS. It is both a beacon of hope and a roadmap to recovery.